Practice Workbook
in
Anatomy and Physiology

A Free Companion to Textbook of Anatomy and Physiology for Nurses

Practice Workbook
in
Anatomy and Physiology

A Free Companion to Textbook of Anatomy and Physiology for Nurses

PR ASHALATHA BSc MBBS MS (Anatomy)
Associate Professor
Department of Anatomy
Government Medical College
Calicut, Kerala, India

Co-author

G DEEPA MBBS MD (Physiology)
Assistant Professor
Department of Physiology
Government Medical College
Thiruvananthapuram, Kerala, India

JAYPEE The Health Sciences Publishers
New Delhi | London | Philadelphia | Panama

Jaypee Brothers Medical Publishers (P) Ltd

Headquarters
Jaypee Brothers Medical Publishers (P) Ltd
4838/24, Ansari Road, Daryaganj
New Delhi 110 002, India
Phone: +91-11-43574357
Fax: +91-11-43574314
Email: jaypee@jaypeebrothers.com

Overseas Offices

J.P. Medical Ltd
83 Victoria Street, London
SW1H 0HW (UK)
Phone: +44 20 3170 8910
Fax: +44 (0)20 3008 6180
Email: info@jpmedpub.com

Jaypee-Highlights Medical Publishers Inc
City of Knowledge, Bld. 237, Clayton
Panama City, Panama
Phone: +1 507-301-0496
Fax: +1 507-301-0499
Email: cservice@jphmedical.com

Jaypee Medical Inc
The Bourse
111 South Independence Mall East
Suite 835, Philadelphia, PA 19106, USA
Phone: +1 267-519-9789
Email: jpmed.us@gmail.com

Jaypee Brothers Medical Publishers (P) Ltd
17/1-B Babar Road, Block-B, Shaymali
Mohammadpur, Dhaka-1207
Bangladesh
Mobile: +08801912003485
Email: jaypeedhaka@gmail.com

Jaypee Brothers Medical Publishers (P) Ltd
Bhotahity, Kathmandu, Nepal
Phone: +977-9741283608
Email: kathmandu@jaypeebrothers.com

Website: www.jaypeebrothers.com
Website: www.jaypeedigital.com

Inquiries for bulk sales may be solicited at: jaypee@jaypeebrothers.com

Practice Workbook in Anatomy and Physiology

First Edition: **2015**

ISBN 978-93-5152-535-6

Printed at Replika Press Pvt. Ltd.

An Insight into the Practice Workbook

Practice Workbook in Anatomy and Physiology is a free companion with the very popular Textbook of Anatomy and Physiology for Nurses by PR Ashalatha and G Deepa. It is an interactive tool that will facilitate structured learning and revision of all the important concepts in every chapter. It has been designed to help in building relevance to the concepts studied.

The important concepts in all the 18 chapters have been covered and the questions are framed in a way to make the learning engaging for the students. Important figure-based questions have been included to aid the nursing students in building concepts and last-minute revision. Long and short answer questions, similar to university examination pattern, have also been included to aid the students in quick revision before the examinations.

For creating an engaging and interesting way of learning, questions on 'match the following', 'true and false', and 'one-word answers' have been included. The answer key to all the questions is included at the end where the page numbers refer to the respective page numbers in the Textbook of Anatomy and Physiology for Nurses. Model test papers from various university examinations have been included at the end of the workbook.

I hope that this new endeavor will be enthusiastically accepted by the students and they will find this workbook as their true companion in the integrated learning of the Anatomy and Physiology.

PR Ashalatha

An Insight into the Practice Workbook

Contents

CHAPTER

1 Introduction to Human Body

Q1 **Figure 1.1 shows various positions of the body. Identify the positions.**

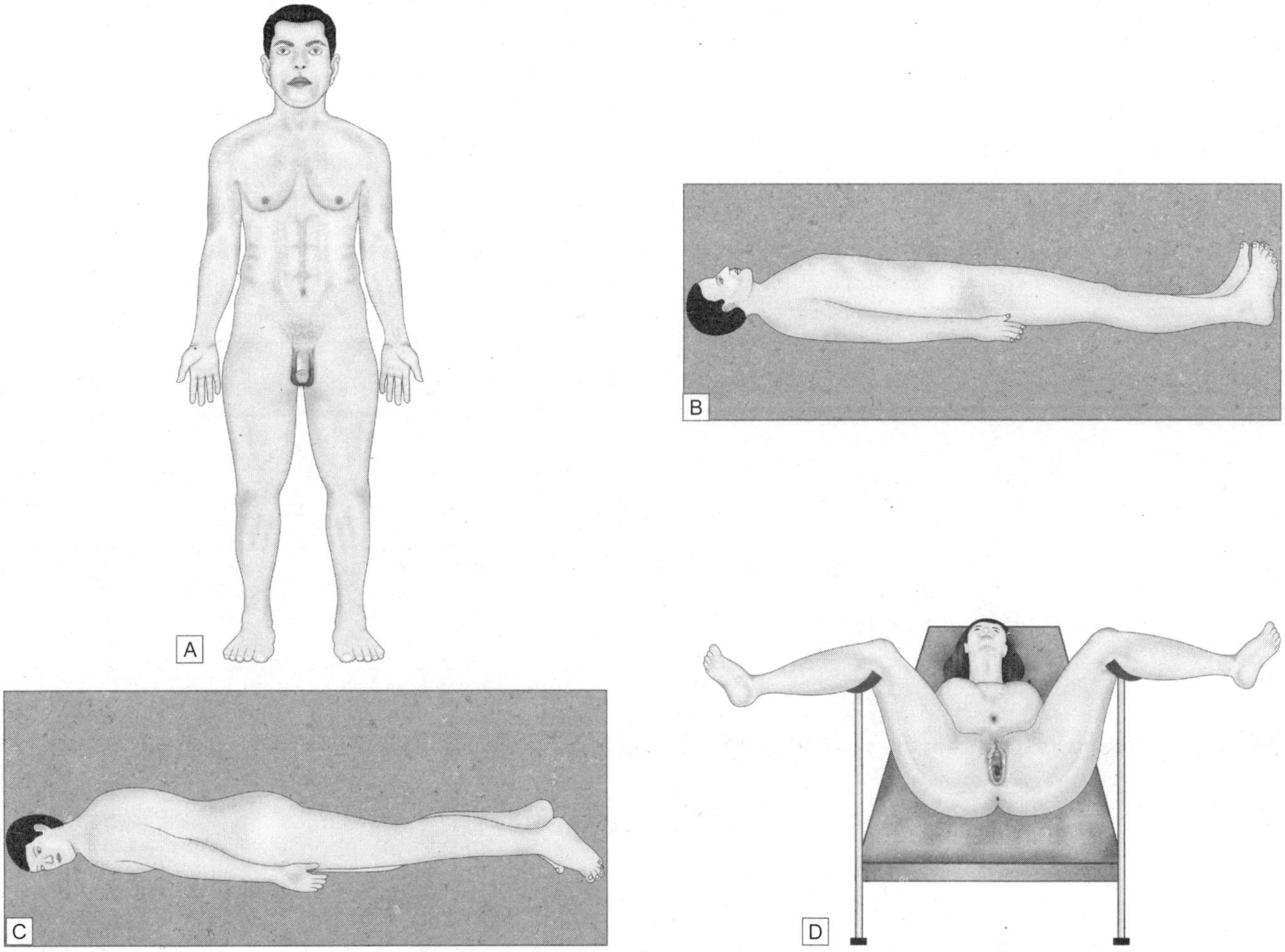

Figs 1.1

A. ____________________

B. ____________________

C. ____________________

D. ____________________

Q2 **What is anatomical position. Give its significance.**

____

____

____

____

____

Q3 **Figure 1.2 shows the various planes of the body. Identify the planes.**

A. ____________________

B. ____________________

C. ____________________

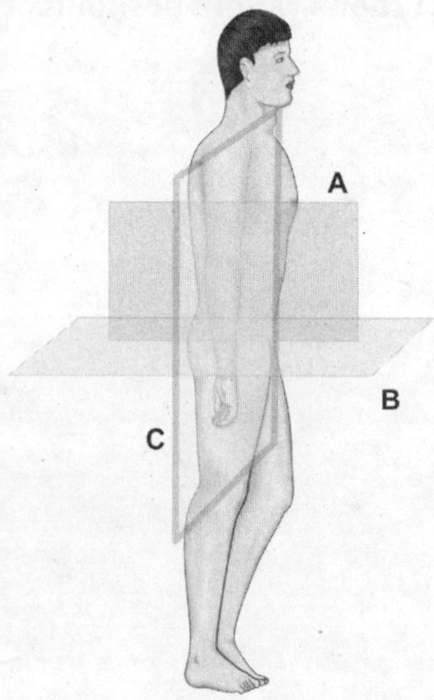

Fig. 1.2

Q4 **Figure 1.3 shows sutures of the skull. Identify the sutures.**

A. ____________________

B. ____________________

C. ____________________

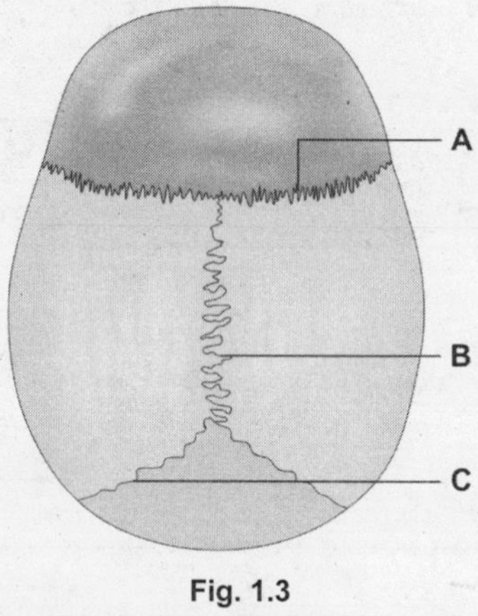

Fig. 1.3

Q5 **Figure 1.4 shows various movements of the body. Identify the movements as indicated in Fig. 1.4.**

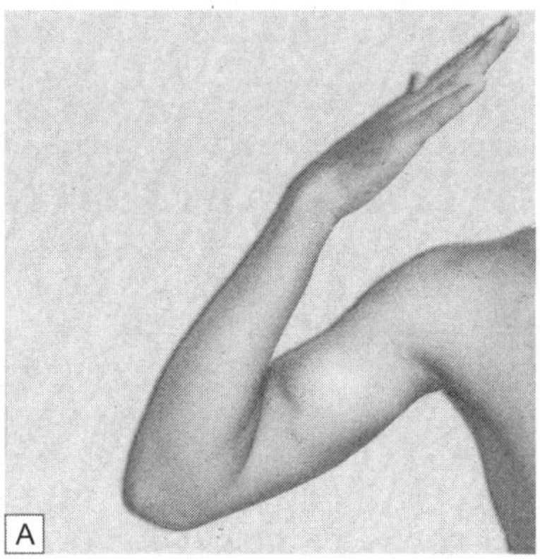

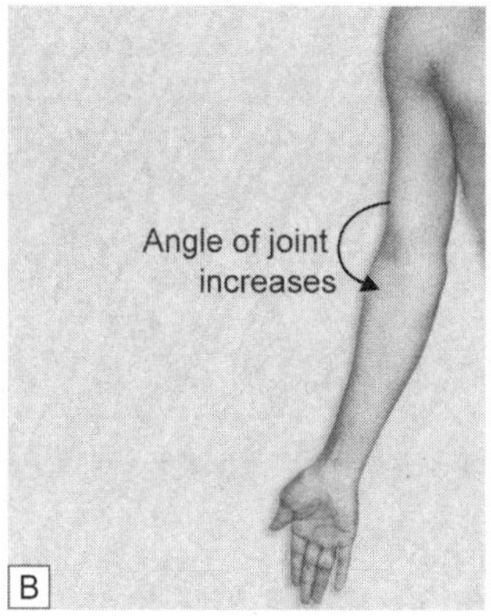

A. ______________________

B. ______________________

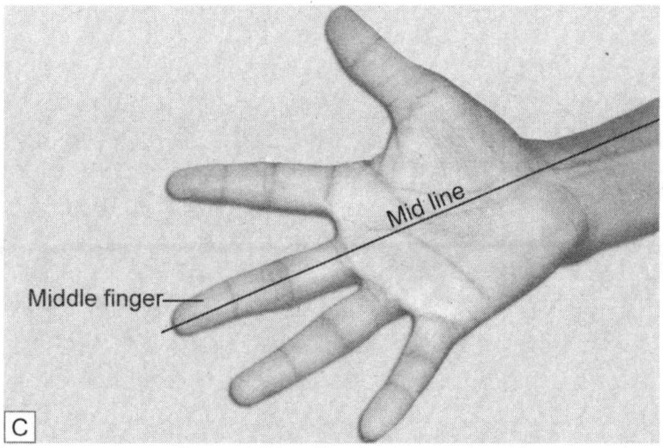

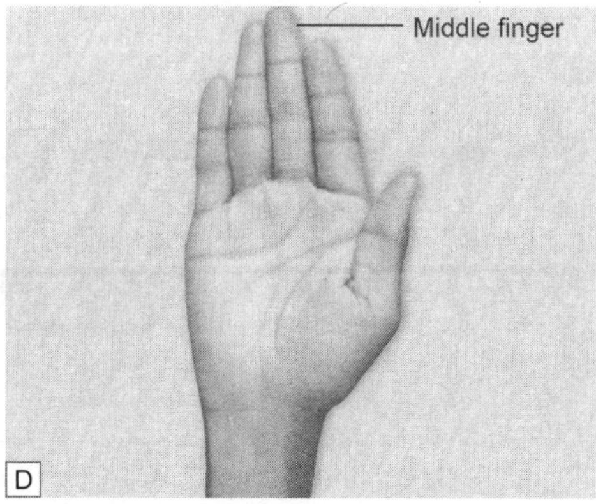

C. ______________________

D. ______________________

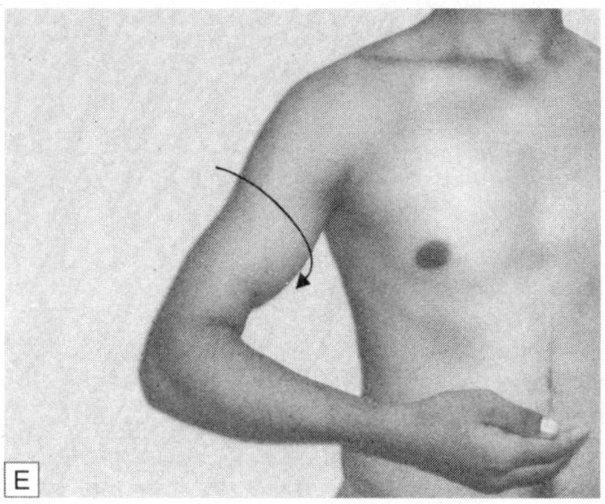

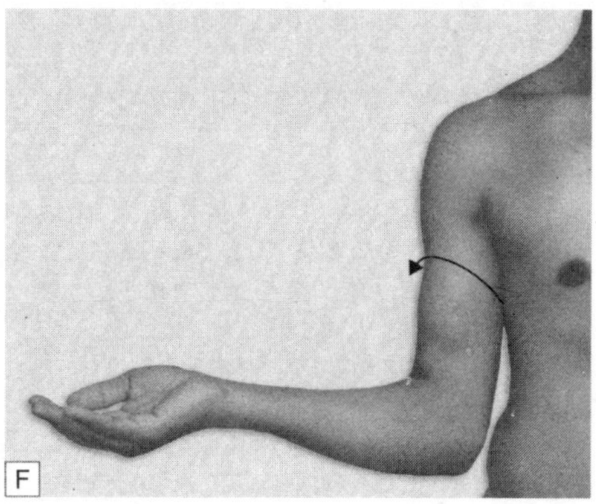

E. ______________________

F. ______________________

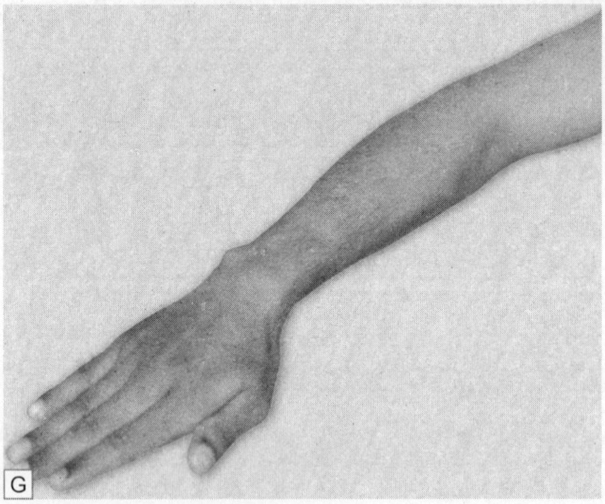

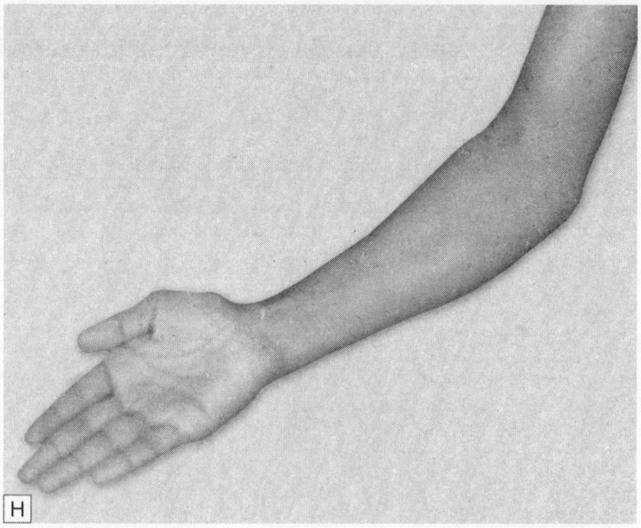

G. ______________________________

H. ______________________________

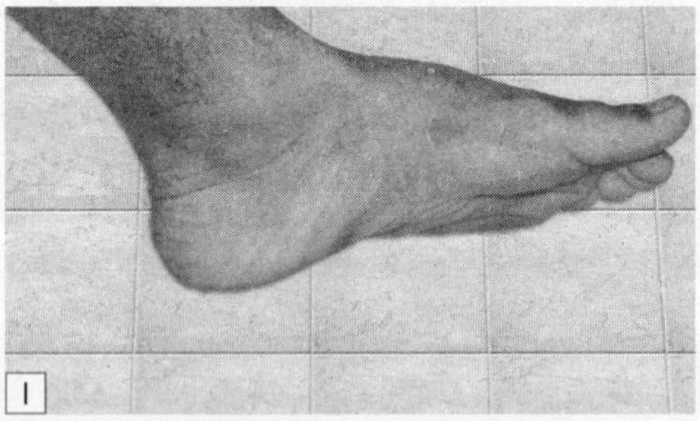

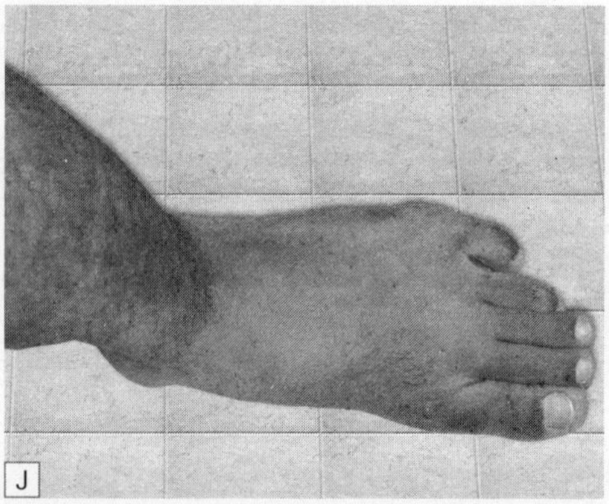

I. ______________________________

J. ______________________________

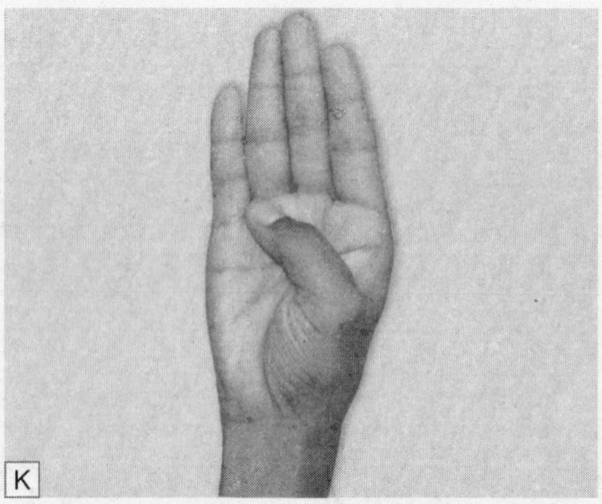

K. ______________________________

Fig. 1.4

Q6 **Figure 1.5 shows various body cavities. Identify the cavities.**

A. ______________________

B. ______________________

C. ______________________

D. ______________________

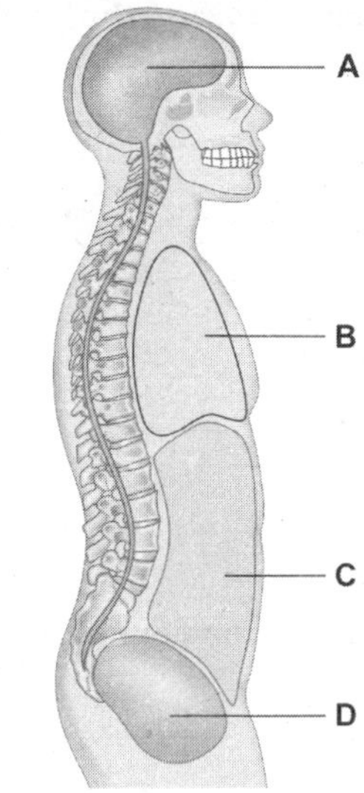

Fig. 1.5

Q7 **Figure 1.6 shows regions of abdominal cavity. Identify the regions.**

A. ______________________

B. ______________________

C. ______________________

D. ______________________

E. ______________________

F. ______________________

G. ______________________

H. ______________________

I. ______________________

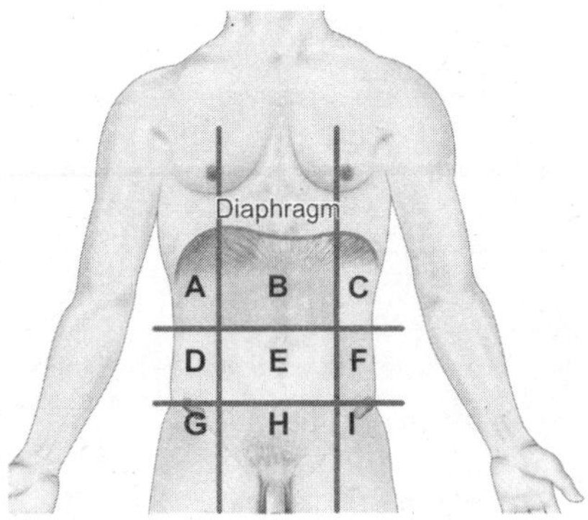

Fig. 1.6

Q8 **Draw a flowchart representing the body water balance.**

Q9 **Draw a flowchart showing the levels of organization of the body.**

Q10 **Define homeostasis and explain positive and negative feedback mechanisms with proper examples.**

Q11 **Define the following terms.**

A. Median plane

B. Sagittal plane

C. Flexion

D. Contralateral

Q12 **Match the following organs with the systems in which they are studied.**

A.	Stomach	1.	Reproductive system
B.	Brain	2.	Urinary system
C.	Heart	3.	Cardiovascular system
D.	Lung	4.	Gastrointestinal system
E.	Uterus	5.	Nervous system
F.	Ureter	6.	Respiratory system

Q13 **Match the following organ with the body cavity in which they are located.**

A.	Lung	1.	Abdominal cavity
B.	Stomach	2.	Pelvic cavity
C.	Brain	3.	Thoracic cavity
D.	Ovaries	4.	Cranial cavity

Q14 **Give one word for.**

A.	Nearer to the head	
B.	Nearer to the feet	
C.	Nearer to the front	
D.	Nearer to the back	
E.	Nearer to the surface	
F.	Nearer to the median plane	
G.	Combined movement of flexion, extension, adduction and abduction in a circular manner	
H.	Movement which causes plantar surface of foot to face inward and downward	
I.	Two structures lying on the same side of body	
J.	The system to which spleen belongs	

Q15 **Match the systems with their functions.**

	System		Function
A.	Integumentary system	1.	Regulation of all body activities
B.	Nervous system	2.	Exchange of gases
C.	Renal system	3.	Production of gametes
D.	Respiratory system	4.	Temperature regulation
E.	Reproductive system	5.	Production, storage and elimination of urine

Q16 **Write True (T) or False (F).**

A.	A person lying face down would be in supine position	
B.	The highest level of structural organization is the system level	
C.	Thyroid and parathyroid glands are included in endocrine system	
D.	Skull and vertebral column are included in appendicular system	
E.	In an average adult, 60% of total body weight is water	
F.	Most of the homeostatic mechanisms of body involve negative feedback system.	

Q17 **Choose the correct answer.**

A. The right ear is ________________ to the right nostril. (medial/lateral)

B. Your lips are ________________ in relation to your nose. (superior/inferior)

C. Your brain is ________________ in relation to your skull. (deep/superficial)

D. To expose brain for surgery, the neurosurgeon would need to cut through the ________________ (thoracic cavity/cranial cavity)

E. An observable or measurable change in the body is called as ________________ (symptom/sign)

CHAPTER

2

Introduction to Chemistry of Life

Q1 **What are dietary fibers. Write in brief their functional significance.**

Q2 **Write in brief the functions of proteins.**

Q3 **What are essential fatty acids.**

Q4 **List the fat soluble vitamins and their deficiency disorders.**

Q5 **Enlist the functions of:**

A. Water

B. Fats

C. Sodium

D. Calcium

E. Vitamin B_{12}

Q6 Write True (T) or False (F).

A.	Daily requirement of carbohydrate is 15–20 g/day	
B.	There are 4 fat soluble vitamins	
C.	Vitamin K is essential for maturation of RBC's	
D.	Proteins supply 9 kcal per gram	
E.	Radioactive isotopes are unstable and release excess energy by emitting radiations	

Q7 Give 3 examples each of:

A. Macrominerals

__________ __________ __________

B. Microminerals

__________ __________ __________

C. Diseases due to deficiency of vitamins

__________ __________ __________

Q8 Give one word for.

A.	Excessive loss of body water	
B.	Linoleic acid, linolenic acid and arachdonic acid	
C.	Deficiency disease of vitamin C	
D.	Elements having same number of protons but different number of neutrons	
E.	Mineral required for formation of bone	

Q9 Match the following.

A.	Polysaccharides	1.	Tryptophan
B.	Dietary fibers	2.	Glycogen
C.	Amino acids	3.	Linoleic acid
D.	Monounsaturated fatty acids	4.	Wheat, Grain
E.	Essential fatty acid	5.	Oleic acid

CHAPTER

3A Organization of Human Body—Cellular Level

Q1 **Define cytology.**

Q2 **Draw and label a eukaryotic cells with its cell organelles.**

Q3 **Figure 3A.1 shows structure of a cell membrane. In the figure identify the structures.**

A. ____________________

B. ____________________

C. ____________________

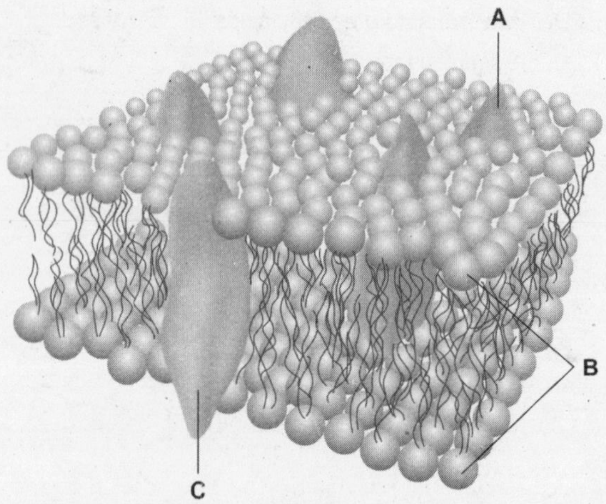

Fig. 3A.1

Q4 **Write the functions of proteins, fats and carbohydrates in the cell membrane.**

Q5 **State the main function of the following organelles.**

A. Smooth endoplasmic reticulum

B. Golgi apparatus

C. Mitochondria

D. Lysosomes

E. Ribosomes

Q6 **Explain with the help of diagrams the process of endocytosis.**

Q7 **Explain with the help of diagrams the process of exocytosis.**

Q8 **Enumerate the following:**

A. The membrane bound organelles

____

B. Structures forming cytoskeleton of cell

____

C. The mechanisms by which substances can be transported passively across the cell membrane

____

D. The major lipids forming the cell membrane

____

E. The parts of a nucleus

____

Q9 **Give one word for.**

A. Power house of the cell

____

B. Structure present in nucleus rich in RNA and proteins

____

C. Natural/programmed cell death

____

D. Structure responsible for the movement of chromosomes during cell division

____

E. Epithelia in which microvilli are not arranged regularly

____

Q10 **Define:**

A. Phagocytosis

____

____

B. Apoptosis

____

____

C. Facilitated diffusion

____

____

D. Active transport

____

____

Q11 Match the following.

A.	Primary active transport	1.	Respiratory epithelium
B.	Cilia	2.	Large contractile protein fibers
C.	Microtubules	3.	Protein synthesis
D.	Mitochondria	4.	Na^+ K^+ ATPase
E.	Rough endoplasmic reticulum	5.	Tricarboxylic acid cycle

Q12 Write True (T) or False (F)

A.	The cell is the smallest functional unit of the body	
B.	Cell membrane is fully permeable	
C.	The hydrophilic portion of phospholipids in the cell membrane face the ECF	
D.	The process by which bacteria are engulfed is called phagocytosis	
E.	Flagella are similar to cilia in structure but smaller than them	
F.	Osmosis is example of active transport.	

CHAPTER

3B

Organization of Human Body—Tissue Level

Q1 **Define tissues and name the four primary tissue of the body.**

____

____

____

____

Q2 **Draw line diagrams of the following in the space provided and give its characteristic.**

	Tissue	Diagram	Characteristics
A.	Simple squamous epithelium		
B.	Simple cuboidal epithelium		
C.	Simple columar epithelium		
D.	Simple tubular gland		
E.	Compound alveolar gland		

Q3 **In Figure 3B.1, identify the type of epithelium represented by:**

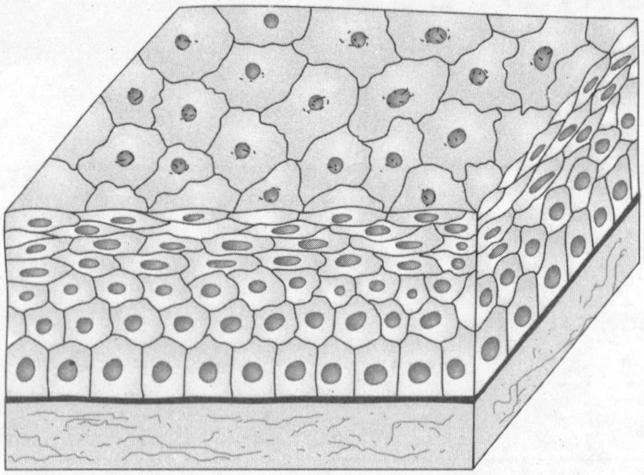

A. ______________________

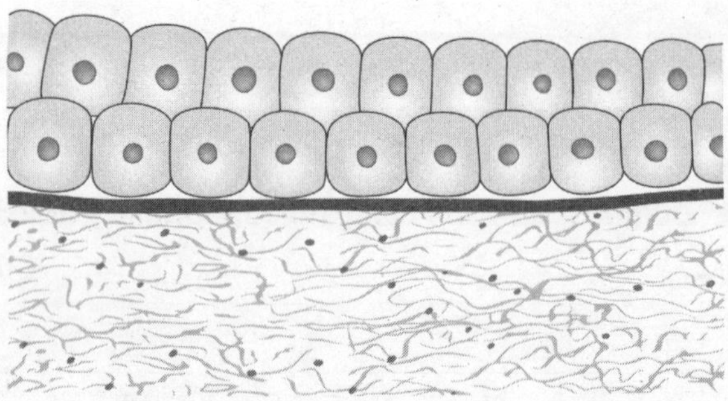

B. ______________________

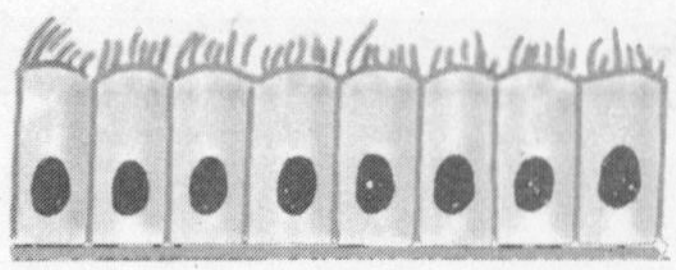

C. ______________________

Fig. 3B.1

Q4 **Figure 3B.2 shows some varieties of glands. Identify the type of glands.**

A. ______________________ B. ______________________

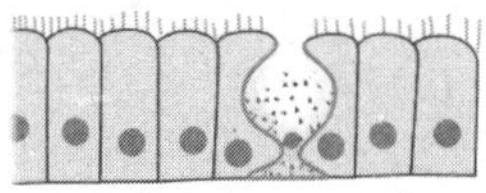

C. ______________________________

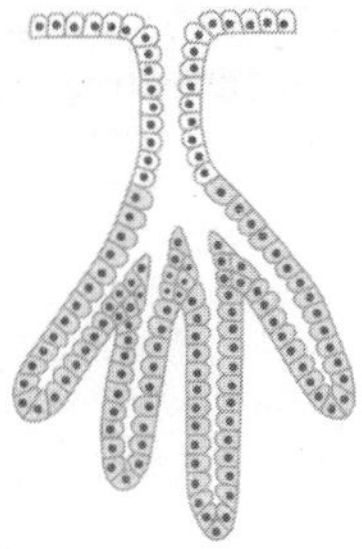

D. ______________________________

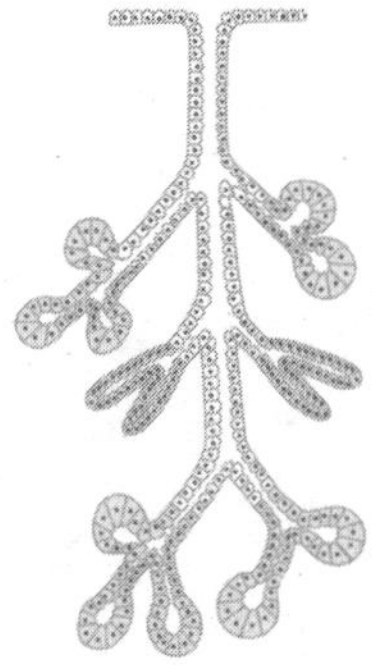

E. ______________________________

Fig. 3B.2

Q5 **Tabulate the differences between serous and mucous glands**

Serous Glands	Mucous Glands

Q6 **Draw and explain what are merocrine, holocrine and apocrine glands**

____

____

____

____

____

____

____

____

____

Q7 **Figure 3B.3 shows components of connective tissue. Identify the structures represented.**

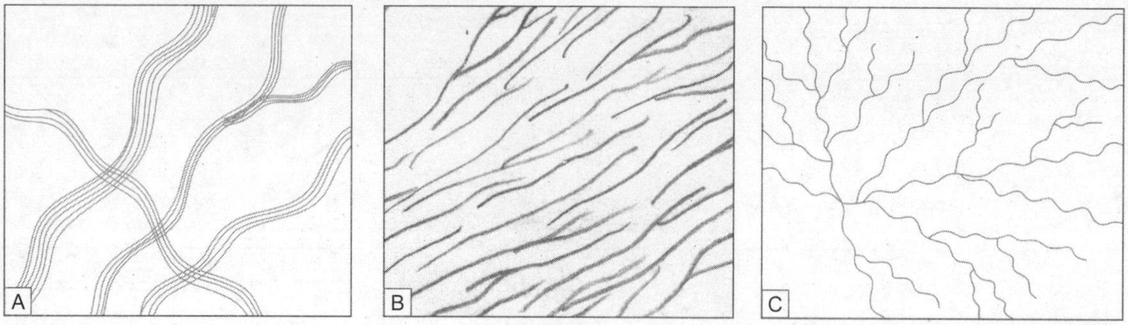

Fig. 3B.3

A. ____________________

B. ____________________

C. ____________________

Q8 **Describe general features of connective tissue.**

Q9 **Name the types of cartilage and write in brief about hyaline cartilage.**

Q10 **Write in brief the functions of:**

A. Epithelial tissue

B. Connective tissue

C. Keratin

Q11 **Enumerate:**

A. The glands on the basis of shape of the secretory unit

B. The parts where ciliated pseudostratified epithelium is found

C. The place where columnar epithelium has goblet cells

D. Types of fibers found in connective tissue

E. Places where adipose tissue is found

Q12 **Match the tissue with the location.**

A.	Dense regular connective	1.	Umbilical cord
B.	Mucoid tissue	2.	Ureter
C.	Transitional epithelium	3.	Dermis of skin
D.	Keratinized stratified squamous epithelium	4.	Thyroid follicles
E.	Cuboidal epithelium	5.	Tendon

Q13 **Write True (T) or False (F).**

A.	Squamous epithelium lining the pleura and peritoneum is called as mesothelium	
B.	Non-ciliated pseudostratified columar epithelium is found in epididymis	
C.	Exocrine glands are ductless glands of the body	
D.	Elastic fibers are called yellow fibers	
E.	Pigment cells are seen in choroid of the eye and skin	

CHAPTER 4

Blood

Q1 Draw flowcharts to show:

A. Composition of blood

B. Steps of erythropoiesis

C. Classification of WBC's

D. Functions of platelets

Q2 **Discuss in brief the physical characteristics of blood.**

Q3 **Discuss in brief the process of hematopoiesis.**

Q4 **Describe the structure and functions of RBC**

Q5 **Write a short note on plasma proteins and their functions.**

Q6 **What is rouleax formation?**

Q7 **Discuss in brief the fate of old RBCs.**

Q8 **What are the functions of hemoglobin in body?**

Q9 **What is ESR? How it can be measured and what is its significance?**

Q10 **Define packed cell volume.**

Q11 **Discuss in brief about hemostasis.**

Q12 **Write a short note on blood transfusion, its indications and hazards.**

Q13 **Explain why it is important to match donor and recepient blood type before giving blood transfusion.**

Q14 **Write a short note on Bombay blood group.**

Q15 **Differentiate between adult and fetal hemoglobin.**

Adult Hemoglobin	Fetal Hemoglobin

Q16 **Define.**

A. Anemia

B. Bleeding time

C. Differential leukocyte count

Q17 **Figure 4.1 shows a sample of anticoagulated blood centrifuged at 300 rpm for 30 minutes. The blood sample gets separated in 3 layers A, B and C. Name these layers.**

A. ______________________

B. ______________________

C. ______________________

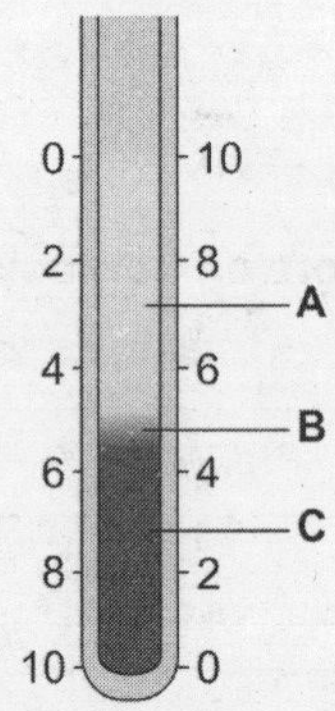

Fig. 4.1

Q18 Write True (T) or False (F)

A.	In adults, the main site of erythropoiesis is red bone marrow	
B.	RBCs are biconvex-shaped cells	
C.	The life span of RBC is 100 days	
D.	Majority of WBCs in body are neutrophils	
E.	In adult hemoglobin, the globin contains 2 α-chains and 2-γ chains	
F.	Liver is called the 'graveyard' of RBCs	
G.	Vitamin K is required for synthesis of clothing factors 2, 7, 9 and 10	
H.	EDTA is an anticoagulant used in laboratories to prevent coagulation of stored blood	
I.	Heparin is an anticoagulant used for therapeutic purposes	
J.	People with blood group O are universal recipients and AB are universal donor	
K.	The most important Rh antigen in D antigen	

Q19 Give one word for.

A.	Ability to generate all mature hematopoietic cells	
B.	Increased RBC count	
C.	Decreased RBC count	
D.	Red pigment found in RBCs	
E.	Leukocytes which have a role in allergy	
F.	Clotting factor 1	
G.	Clotting factor 2	
H.	Substances which prevent clotting	

Q20 Give normal values of:

A.	pH of blood	
B.	Albumin–globulin ratio	
C.	RBC count	
D.	Hemoglobin levels	
E.	PCV	
F.	TLC	
G.	Platelet count	

CHAPTER

5

Lymphatic System

Q1

Draw a flowchart to show the composition of lymph.

Q2

Name the places in body where lymph capillaries are absent.

____

____

Q3

Write short note on thoracic duct.

____

____

____

____

____

____

Q4

Figure 5.1 shows areas of body drained by thoracic duct and right lymphatic duct. In the figure, A and B represent.

A. ____

B. ____

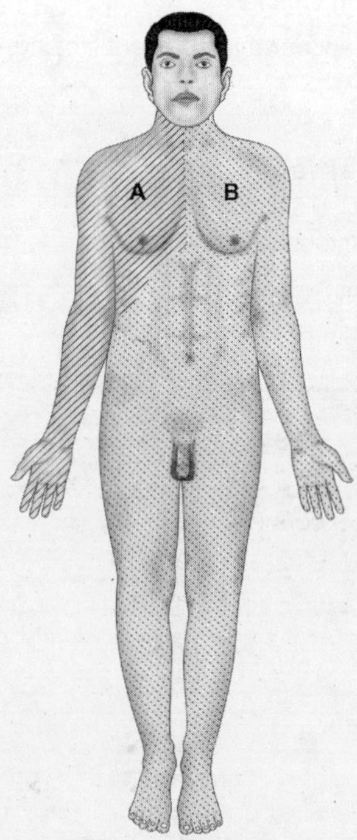

Fig. 5.1

Q5 **Write a short note on lymph nodes.**

Q6 **Draw a diagram to show organs related to spleen.**

Q7 **Write a short note on functions of spleen.**

Q8 **Discuss in brief the blood supply of tonsils along with diagram.**

Q9 **Name the following**

A. Structures forming bed of tonsil

B. Deep group of cervical lymph nodes

C. Lymph nodes draining the breast

D. Lymph nodes draining the lower limb

E. Structures entering and leaving spleen at hilum

F. Collection of lymphoid tissue present at the entrance of alimentary tract

G. Lymph nodes draining the tonsils

H. The condition of spleen enlargement

I. Organ called as "graveyard" of RBCs

Q10 **Explain the formation and flow of lymph.**

Q11 **Write True (T) or False (F).**

A.	The tissue fluid that enters lymphatic system is called plasma	
B.	Lymphocytes are most abundant cells of lymph	
C.	The inner lining of lymph capillaries is called as endothelium	
D.	Large lymphatic vessels are similar to veins as they have numerous valves	
E.	Retrograde flow can take place in lymphatic vessels	
F.	Tonsils and lymph nodes are examples of primary lymphoid organs	
G.	White pulp and red pulp are seen in tonsils	
H.	The size of thymus increases throughout life	

CHAPTER

6

Resistance and Immunity

Q1 **Define and classify immunity.**

Q2 **Discuss in brief innate immunity.**

Q3 **Write a short note on:**

A. Immunoglobulins

B. MHC

C. Reticuloendothelial system

Q4 **Draw a flowchart to show functions of antibodies.**

Q5 **Outline the steps in**

A. Cell-mediated immunity

B. Antibody-mediated immunity

Q6 **Compare cell-mediated and antibody-mediated immunity.**

Cell-mediated immunity	Antibody-mediated immunity

Q7 **Write True (T) or False (F):**

A	Lysozymes and interferons are examples of natural antimicrobial substances present in body.	
B	Natural killer cells do not have B or T cell markers	
C	Humoral immunity is mediated by T-lymphocytes	
D	Most abundant immunoglobulin present in saliva and sweat is IgA	
E	IgM antibodies can cross the placenta	
F	T-lymphocytes can recognize only those antigens which are presented with MHC.	
G	Natural killer cells are a part of innate immunity	

CHAPTER

7

Nervous System

Q1 **Figure 7.1 shows anatomical divisions of the nervous system. Identify the structures.**

A. ____________________

B. ____________________

C. ____________________

D. ____________________

E. ____________________

F. ____________________

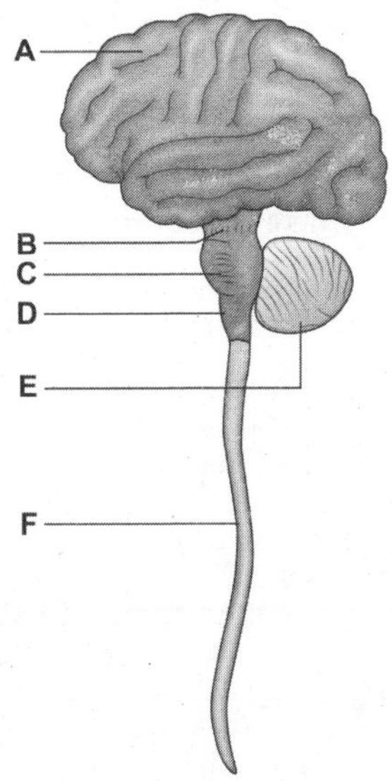

Fig. 7.1

Q2 **Figure 7.2 shows Structure of a neuron. Identify the structures.**

A. ____________________

B. ____________________

C. ____________________

D. ____________________

E. ____________________

F. ____________________

G. ____________________

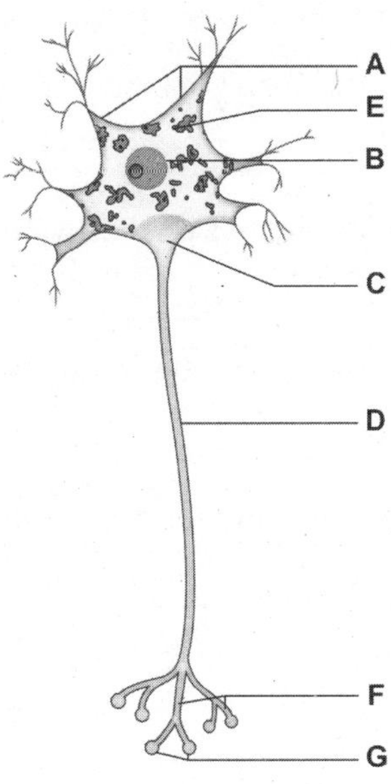

Fig. 7.2

Q3 **Figure 7.3 shows structure of a typical chemical synapse. Identify the structures.**

A. ______________________

B. ______________________

C. ______________________

D. ______________________

E. ______________________

F. ______________________

G. ______________________

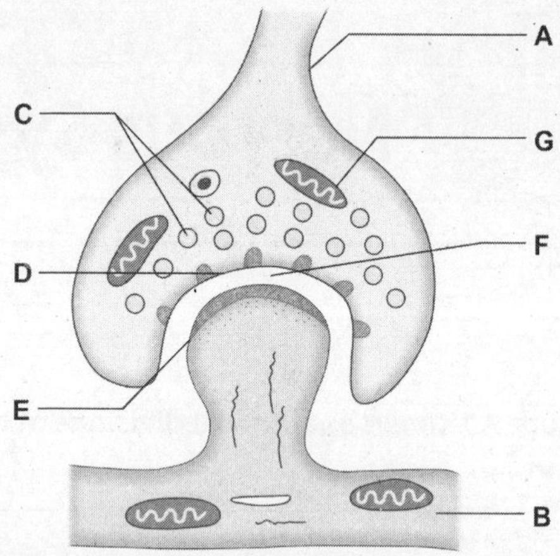

Fig. 7.3

Q4 **Figure 7.4 shows phases of action potential in a neuron. Identify the phases of action potential:**

A. ______________________

B. ______________________

C. ______________________

D. ______________________

E. ______________________

F. ______________________

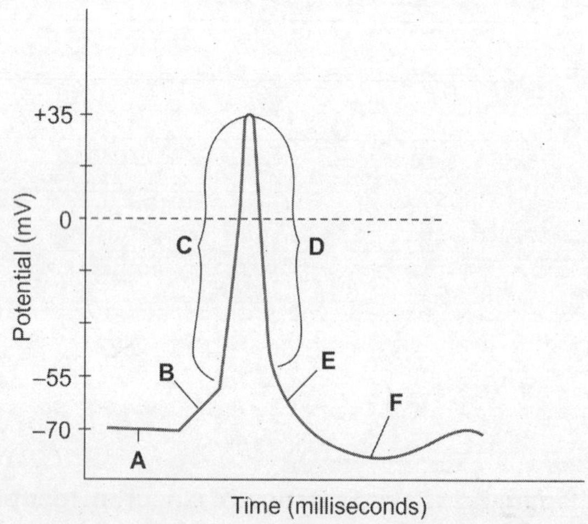

Fig. 7.4

In the figure:

A. What is the firing level shown for the neuron

____

B. What is the peak value shown for the neuron

____

C. Depolarization of neuron is attributed to

____

D. Repolarization of neuron is attributed to

____

Q5 **Figure 7.5 shows the ventricular system of the brain. Identify the structure.**

A. ______________________

B. ______________________

C. ______________________

D. ______________________

E. ______________________

F. ______________________

G. ______________________

H. ______________________

I. ______________________

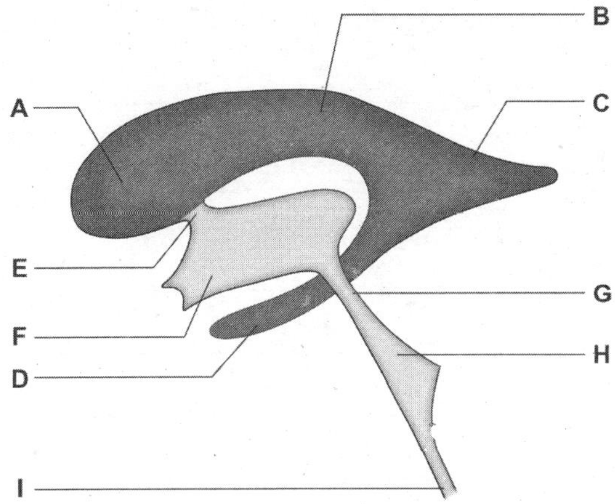

Fig. 7.5

Q6 **Figure 7.6 shows superior view of cerebrum. Identify the structures indicated.**

A. ______________________

B. ______________________

C. ______________________

D. ______________________

E. ______________________

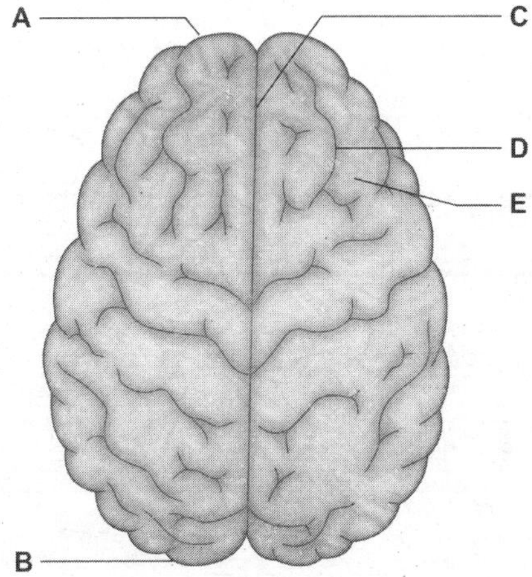

Fig. 7.6

Q7 **Figure 7.7 shows lateral aspect of cerebral hemisphere.**

Identify the poles:

A. ______________________

B. ______________________

C. ______________________

Identify the sulci:

1. ______________________

2. ______________________

3. ______________________

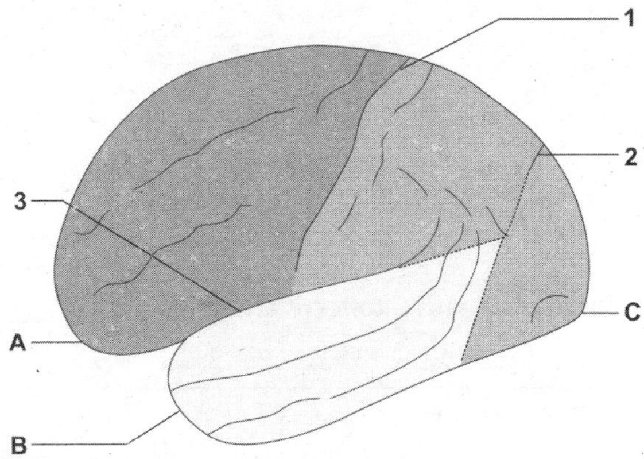

Fig. 7.7

Q8 **Figure 7.8 shows circle of Willis.**

Identify the arteries:

A. ______________________

B. ______________________

C. ______________________

D. ______________________

E. ______________________

F. ______________________

G. ______________________

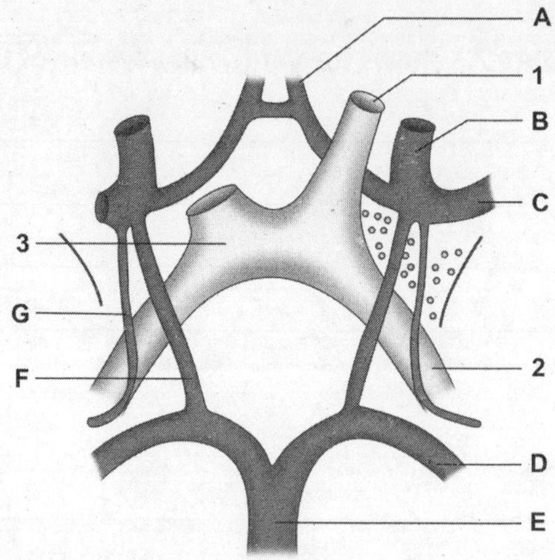

Fig. 7.8

What do structures 1, 2, 3 represent:

1. ______________________

2. ______________________

3. ______________________

Q9 **Figure 7.9 shows internal capsule and its relations in the figure label the parts of internal capsule.**

Identify structures:

A. ______________________

B. ______________________

C. ______________________

D. ______________________

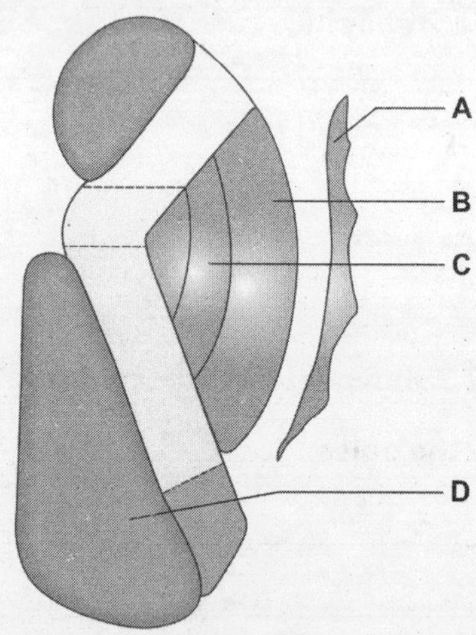

Fig. 7.9

What are B and C collectively called as:

____

Q10 **Figure 7.10 shows ventral aspect of Brainstem. Mark midbrain, pons, medulla and spinal cord in the figure. Identify structures.**

A. ______________________

B. ______________________

C. ______________________

D. ______________________

E. ______________________

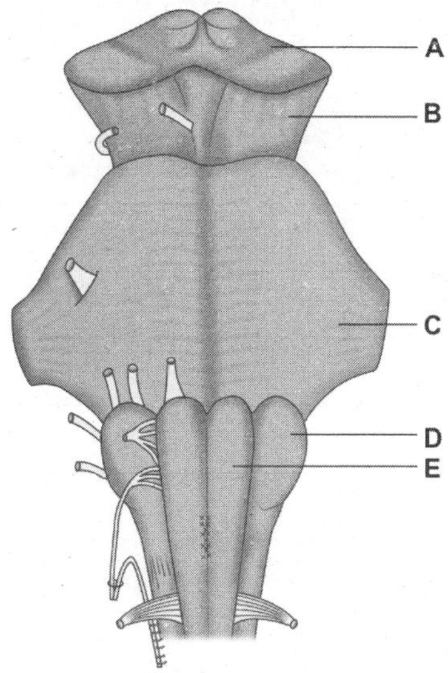

Fig. 7.10

Q11 **Figure 7.11 shows T.S. of spinal cord. Identify the structures.**

A. ______________________

B. ______________________

C. ______________________

D. ______________________

E. ______________________

F. ______________________

G. ______________________

H. ______________________

I. ______________________

J. ______________________

K. ______________________

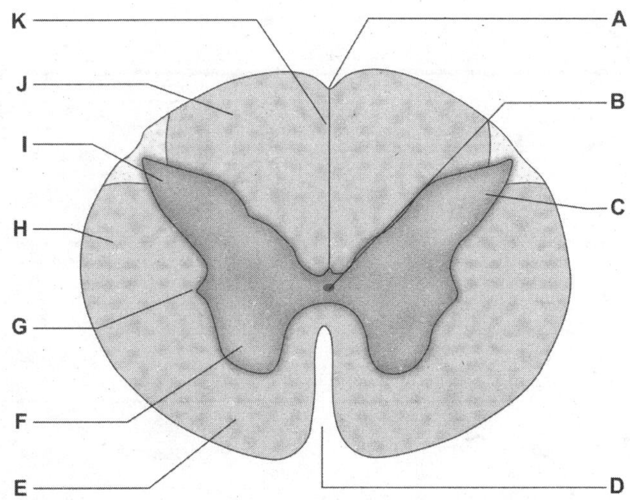

Fig. 7.11

How is the arrangement of grey and white matter in spinal cord different from that of brain.

____

____

____

Q12 **Figure 7.12 shows the synapses of autonomic nervous system. In figure identify the neurotransmitter released in synapse**

A. ____________________

B. ____________________

C. ____________________

D. ____________________

E. ____________________

F. ____________________

G. ____________________

H. ____________________

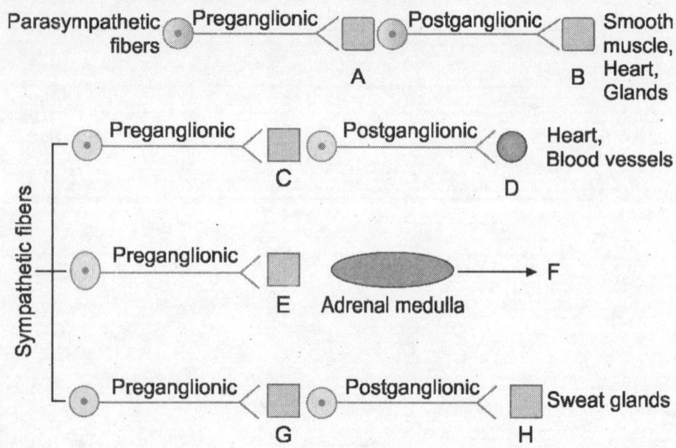

Fig. 7.12

Q13 **Figure 7.13 shows ventral aspect of brain stem. Draw the origin of all cranial nerves arising from ventral aspect. name the cranial nerve which arises from dorsal aspect of brain.**

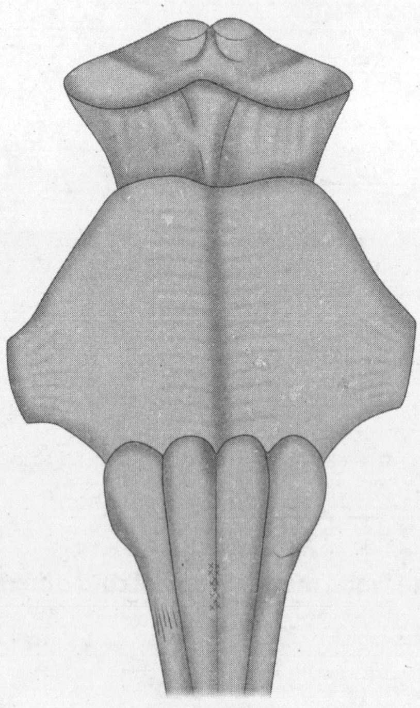

Fig. 7.13

Q14 Draw an algorithm showing classification of synapses.

Q15 Draw and label parts of lateral ventricle.

Q16 Draw and label major functional areas of brain.

Q17 **Draw and label pathway of spinothalamic tract.**

Q18 **Draw and label pathway of pyramidal tract.**

Q19 **Draw the types of neurons based on polarity.**

Q20 **Draw a simple reflex arc.**

Q21 **Draw a flowchart to show divisions of nervous system.**

Q22 **Discuss briefly the structure of neuron.**

Q23 **Discuss briefly the structure of synapse.**

Q24 **Define**

A. Absolute refractory period

B. Synapse

C. Reticular formation

D. Spinal segment

E. Reflex

F. Rigidity

Q25 **Write in brief the functions of**

A. Hypothalamus

B. Cerebellum

C. Pyramidal tract

D. Cerebrum

E. Thalamus

Q26 Write short notes on:

A. Degeneration of nerve fibers

B. Cerebrospinal fluid

C. Blood brain barrier

D. Internal capsule

E. Circle of Willis

F. Babinski's sign

G. Carpal tunnel syndrome

H. Referred pain

Q27 **Differentiate between**

A. Upper motor neuron lesion and lower motor neuron lesion

Upper motor neuron lesion	Lower motor neuron lesion

B. Pyramidal and Extrapyramidal tract lesion

Pyramidal tract lesion	Extrapyramidal tract lesion

Q28

Enumerate

A. Central neuroglial cells

B. Meninges from outside to inside

C. Two sites where choroid plexus is present

D. Two areas where blood brain barrier is absent

E. Parts of hind brain

F. Types of fibers present in white matter of cerebrum

G. Nuclei included in basal nuclei (ganglia)

H. The centres in hypothalamus for regulation of hunger and food intake

I. The branches of internal carotid artery supplying the brain

J. The ascending tracts of spinal cord

K. The nerve roots taking part in the formation of brachial plexus

____

L. The nerve roots taking part in the formation of lumbar plexus

____

Q29 Give one word for:

A. The cells forming myelin sheath in CNS

____

B. The cells forming myelin sheath in PNS

____

C. The part of nerve fiber between two consecutive nodes of Ranvier

____

D. The mechanism of conduction of action potential in myelinated nerve fiber

____

E. Ventricle situated between the right and left thalamus

____

F. The structure responsible for the secretion of CSF

____

G. Midbrain, pons and medulla together

____

H. The peduncle connecting pons to cerebellum

____

I. Series of rapid and repeated involuntary jerky movements which occur while eliciting a deep reflex

____

J. Loss of sensory perception

____

Q30 Match the following:

	Nerve		Name
A.	IV	1.	Facial nerve
B.	VII	2.	Accessory nerve
C.	V	3.	Trochlear nerve
D.	VIII	4.	Trigeminal nerve
E.	XI	5.	Vestibulocochlear nerve

Q31

Match the following:

	Area		Broadmann number
A.	Primary motor area	1.	Area 44, 45
B.	Motor speech area	2.	Area 17
C.	Somatosensory area I	3.	Area 4
D.	Primary auditory area	4.	Area 3, 1, 2
E.	Primary visual area	5.	Area 41, 42

CHAPTER

8A Musculoskeletal System— Muscular System

Q1 **Figure 8A.1 shows connective tissue present in relation to skeletal muscle. Identify A, B and C.**

A. ______________________________

B. ______________________________

C. ______________________________

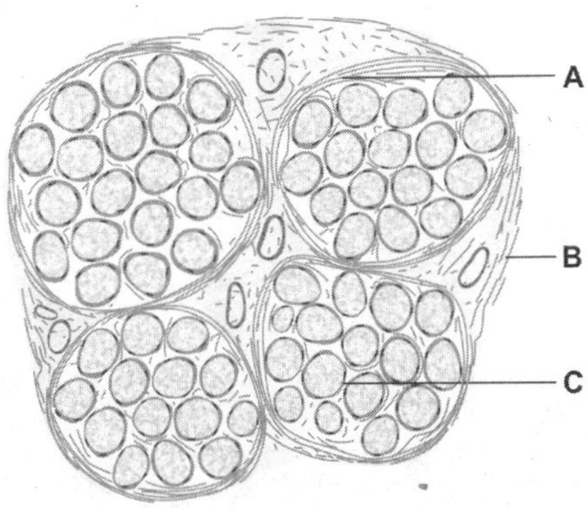

Fig. 8A.1

Q2 **Figure 8A.2 shows a myofibril. Identify the zones/bands represented by A, B, C, D and E.**

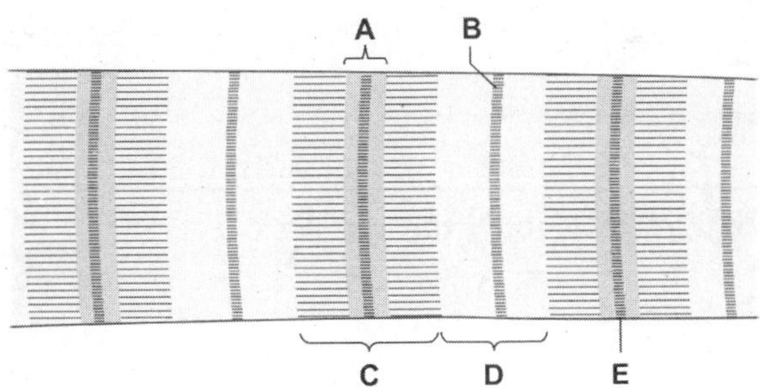

Fig. 8A.2

A. ______________________________

B. ______________________________

C. ______________________________

D. ______________________________

E. ______________________________

Q3 **Figure 8A.3 shows a neuromuscular junction. Identify the parts.**

A. ____________________

B. ____________________

C. ____________________

D. ____________________

E. ____________________

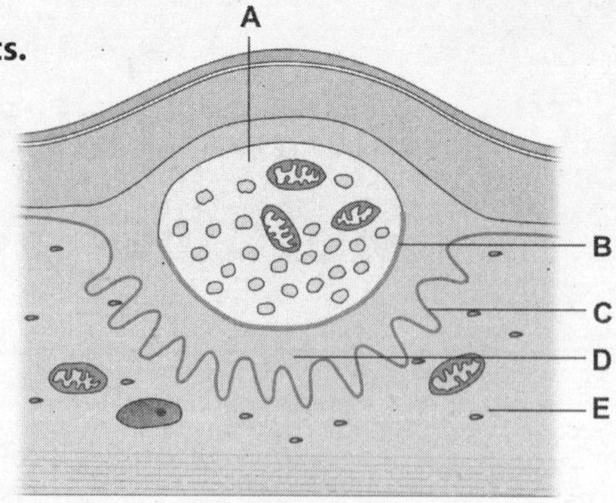

Fig. 8A.3

Q4 **Figure 8A.4 shows cross-section of muscles. Identify the type of muscle.**

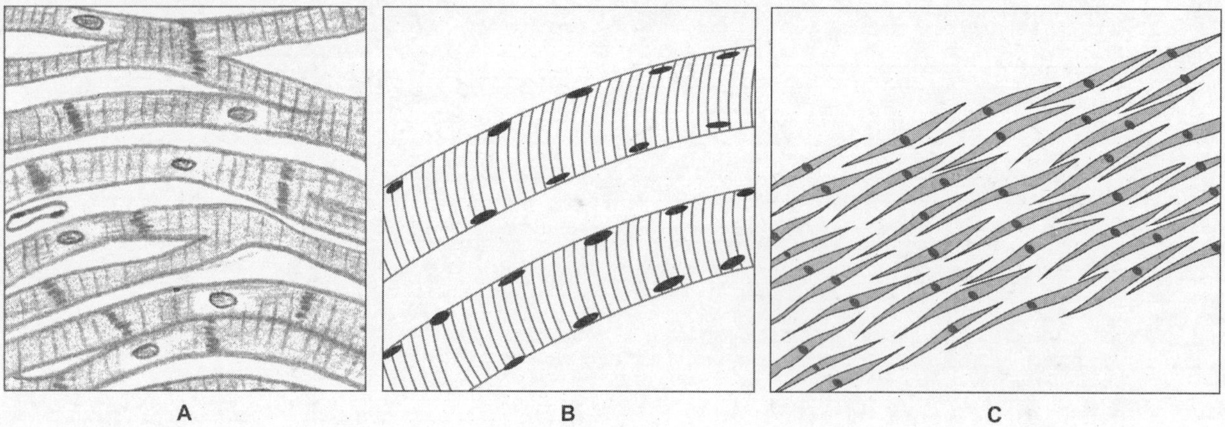

Fig. 8A.4

A. ____________________

B. ____________________

C. ____________________

Q5 **Figure 8A.5 shows muscles of the face. Identify the muscles.**

A. ____________________

B. ____________________

C. ____________________

D. ____________________

E. ____________________

F. ____________________

G. ____________________

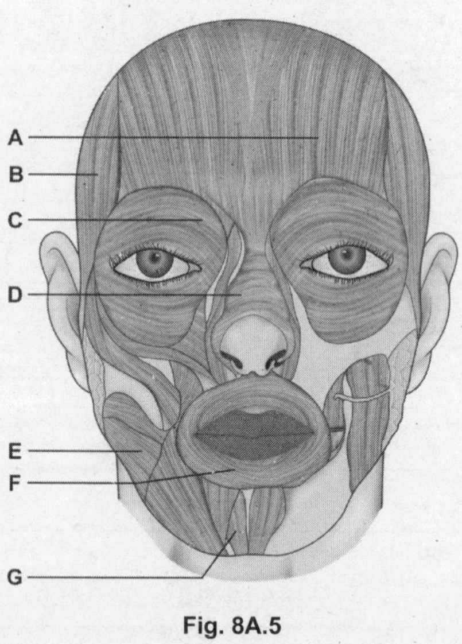

Fig. 8A.5

Q6 **Figure 8A.6 shows muscles of the neck. Identify the muscles.**

A. ______________________

B. ______________________

C. ______________________

D. ______________________

E. ______________________

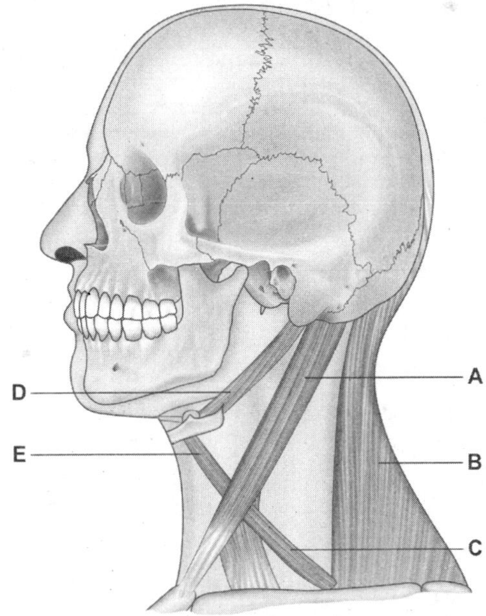

Fig. 8A.6

Q7 **Figure 8A.7 shows anterior aspect of muscles of arm. Identify the muscles.**

A. ______________________

B. ______________________

C. ______________________

D. ______________________

E. ______________________

F. ______________________

G. ______________________

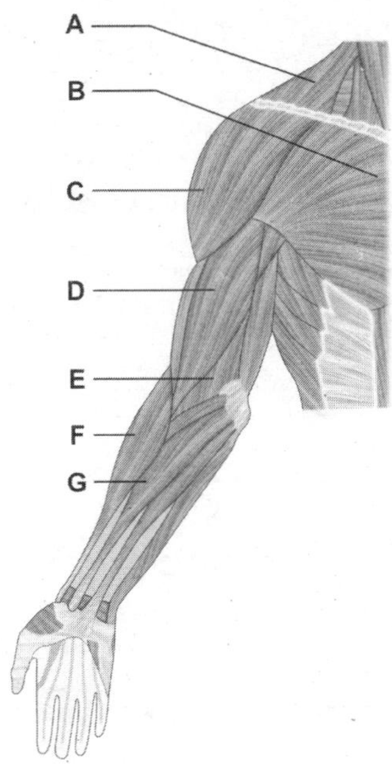

Fig. 8A.7

Q8 **Figure 8A.8 shows important muscles of lower limb (posterior aspect). Identify the muscles. Which structure is represented by F.**

A. ______________________

B. ______________________

C. ______________________

D. ______________________

E. ______________________

F. ______________________

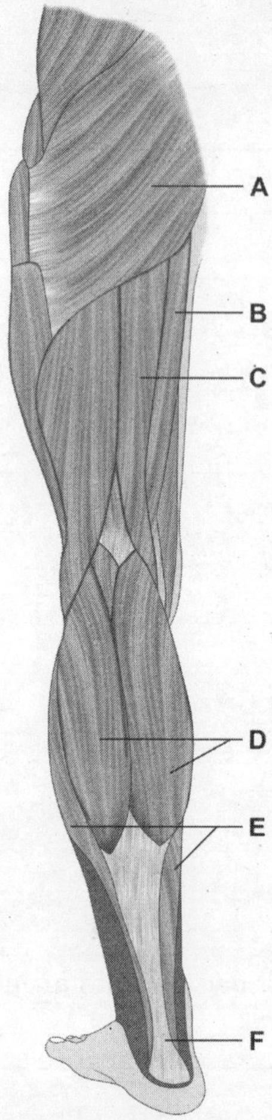

Fig. 8A.8

Q9 **Write in brief the characteristics of skeletal muscle.**

____

____

____

____

Q10 **Discuss briefly about neuromuscular junction**

____

____

____

____

Q11 **Define the following terms:**

A. Isometric contraction

____

____

B. Motor unit

____

____

C. Sarcomere

____

____

D. Muscle tone

____

____

Q12 **Name the three major foramina present in diaphragm and the structures passing through them.**

____

____

____

____

Q13 **Differentiate between**

A. Skeletal muscles and cardiac muscles

Skeletal muscle	Cardiac muscle

B. Slow fibers and fast fibers

Slow fiber	Fast fiber

Q14 **Give the origin, insertion, nerve supply and action of following muscles**

Muscle	Origin	Insertion	Nerve supply	Action
Occipitofrontalis				
Sternocleidomastoid				
Gastrocnemius				
Psoas major				
Deltoid				
Pectoralis major				
Latissimus dorsi				
Sartorius				

Q15 **Name the following:**

A. Muscles forming posterior abdominal wall

B. Muscles attaching humerus to chest wall

C. Muscles of anterior compartment of arm

D. Three gluteal muscles.

E. Adductor muscles of thigh

F. Muscles of mastication

Q16 **Write short notes on**

A. Hamstrings muscles

B. Myasthenia gravis

C. Achilles tendon

D. Inguinal canal

Q17 **Draw a neatly labeled diagram of pelvic diaphragm.**

Q18 **Match the following:**

	Muscle		Region
A.	Sternocleidomastoid	1.	Upper limb
B.	Rectus abdominis	2.	Lower limb
C.	Psoas major	3.	Face
D.	Deltoid	4.	Neck
E.	Gluteus maximus	5.	Anterior abdominal wall
F.	Occipitofrontalis	6.	Thorax
G.	Intercostal muscle	7.	Posterior abdominal wall

Q19 **True or False**

A.	Intercalated discs are present in skeletal muscles	
B.	Sarcoplasmic reticulum is another name for endoplasmic reticulum present in muscles	
C.	The resting membrane potential of muscles is –90 mV	
D.	Motor supply to diaphragm is by phrenic nerve	
E.	Biceps are supplied by musculocutaneous nerve	
F.	Triceps are the main muscles which bring about extension of elbow joint	
G.	Quadriceps femoris and sartorious are supplied by femoral nerve	
H.	Adductor magnus is the largest muscle of adductor compartment of leg	

CHAPTER

8B

Musculoskeletal System—Skeletal System

Q1 **Draw a flowchart to show the composition of bone**

Q2 **Figure 8B.1 shows human skeleton. Name the bones shown in the figure.**

A. ______

B. ______

C. ______

D. ______

E. ______

F. ______

G. ______

H. ______

I. ______

J. ______

K. ______

L. ______

M. ______

O. ______

P. ______

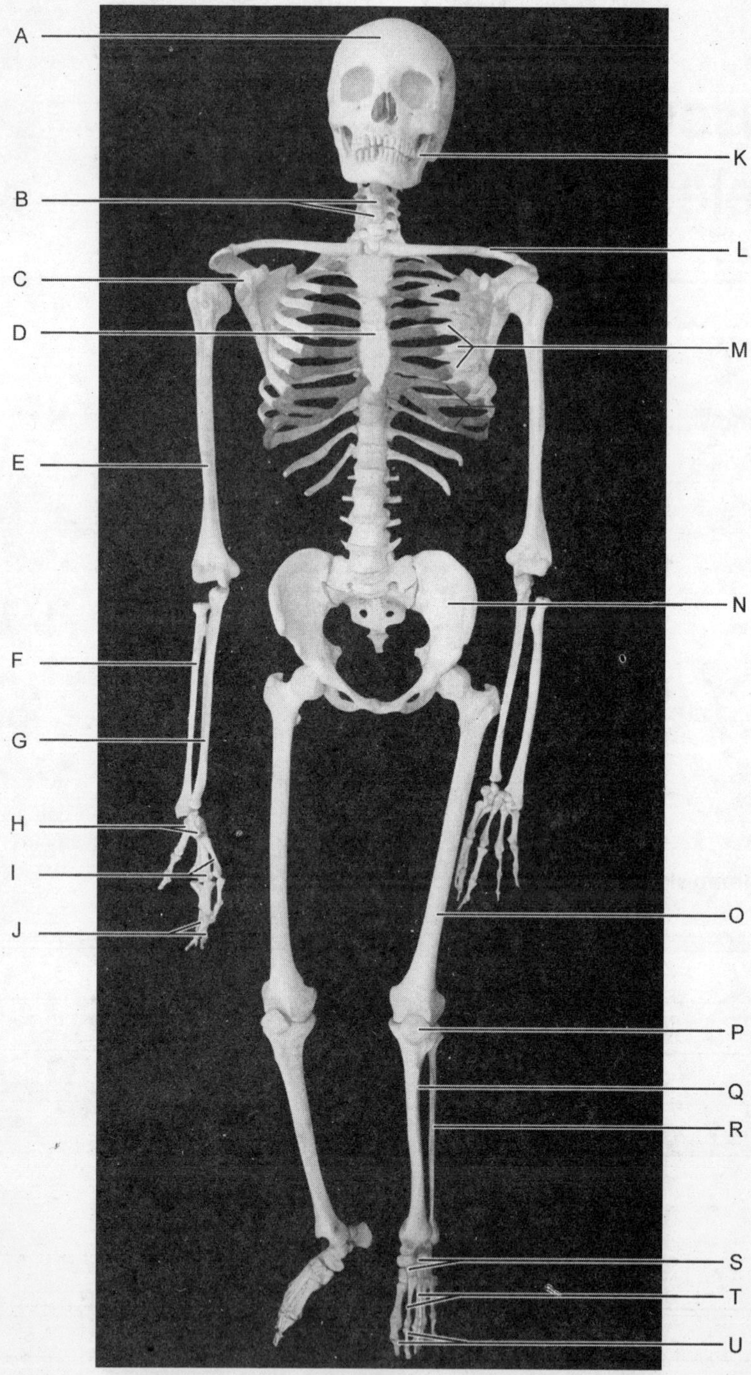

Fig. 8B.1

Q. ____________________

R. ____________________

S. ____________________

T. ____________________

U. ____________________

Q3 **Figure 8B.2 shows norma verticalis of skull. Identify the sutures shown. What are the points shown by D and E called.**

A. ____________________

B. ____________________

C. ____________________

D. ____________________

E. ____________________

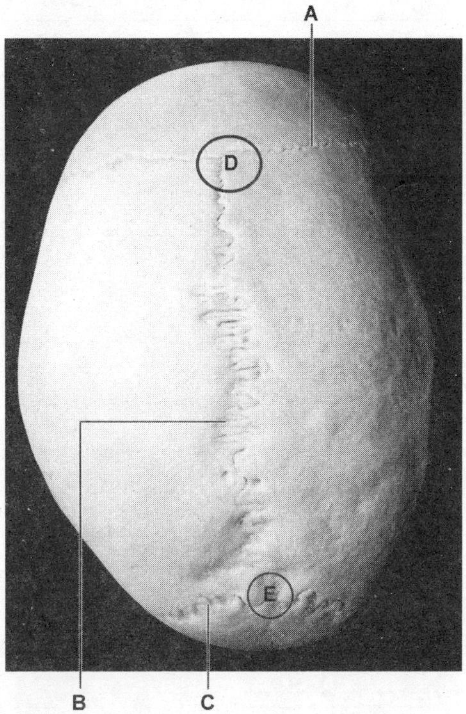

Fig. 8B.2

Q4 **Figure 8B.3 shows thoracic cage. Identify the structures shown.**

A. ____________________

B. ____________________

C. ____________________

D. ____________________

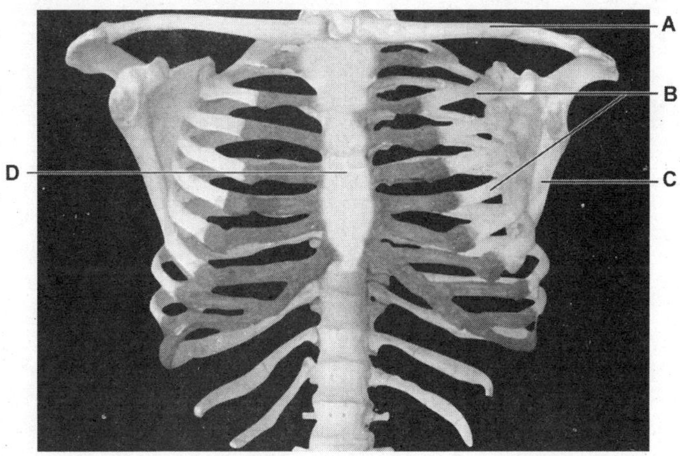

Fig. 8B.3

Q5 **Figure 8B.4 shows parts of a typical vertebra. Identify the structures.**

A. ____________________

B. ____________________

C. ____________________

D. ____________________

E. ____________________

F. ____________________

G. ____________________

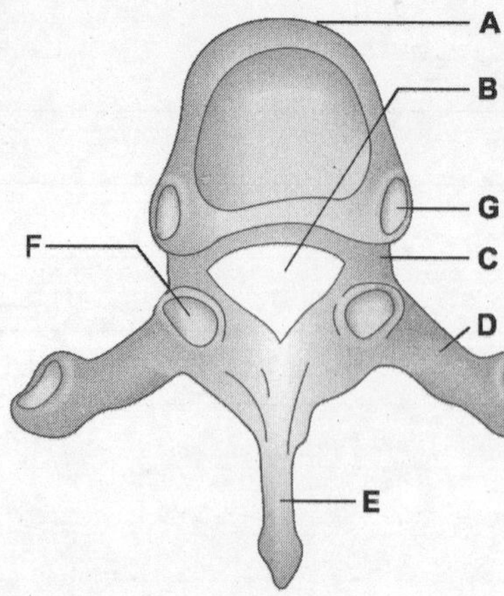

Fig. 8B.4

Q6 **Discuss briefly the Haversian system of bone.**

____

____

____

____

____

____

Q7 **Explain with the help of diagram, the parts of long bone.**

____

____

____

____

____

____

____

____

____

____

____

Q8 **Discuss briefly the functions of bone**

Q9 **How does a newborn skull differs from an adult skull.**

Q10 **How many vertebrae are present in vertebral column. What are primary and secondary curvatures.**

Q11 **Name the following:**

A. The cells present in bone

B. Two flatbones present in body

C. The bones which make up axial skeleton

D. The two mechanisms of bone formation

E. The five main bones which form the upper limb

F. Contents of sacral canal

G. Muscles attached to the clavicle bone

H. The bones which form the pelvic girdle

I. The unpaired bones of face

J. The structures passing through foramen magnum

K. The atypical ribs

Q12 Write short notes on:

A. Sesamoid bone

B. Cancellous bones

C. Metaphysis

D. Typical vertebra

E. Identifying features of cervical vertebra

F. True pelvis and false pelvis

____

____

____

Q13 Write True (T) or False (F):

A.	All the newly formed bones are of lamellar variety	
B.	Another name for cancellous bones is spongy bones	
C.	Long bones ossify in cartilage.	
D.	A total of 206 bones constitute adult human skeleton	
E.	Skull is made of 26 bones.	
F.	There are a total of 8 carpal bones and 5 metacarpal bones in each upper limb.	
G.	Most common variety of pelvis is android pelvis	
H.	Face has 14 bones.	
I.	Patella is the largest sesamoid bone in the body	
J.	Foramen magnum is seen in lateral part of skull.	
K.	Vertebral artery passes through foramen transversarium of all cervical vertebrae except C 7.	
L.	Most common site of fracture of clavicle is the junction of medial one-third and lateral two–thirds.	

Q14 Match the following parts of bones with their respective bones.

A.	Manubrium	1.	Scapula
B.	Odontoid process	2.	Ulna
C.	Acromion process	3.	Sternum
D.	Olecranon process	4.	Hip bone
E.	Obturator foramen	5.	Axis vertebra

Q15 Give one word for:

A.	The point where sagittal and lambdoid sutures meet	
B.	Bone forming the lower jaw	
C.	First cervical vertebra	
D.	Oval foramen present in each transverse process of a typical cervical vertebra	
E.	Tail bone	

Q16 **Match the following:**

	Bones		Part of body
A.	Radius	1.	Lower limb
B.	Carpal bones	2.	Knee
C.	Atlas	3.	Upper limb
D.	Fibula	4.	Hand
E.	Patella	5.	Vertebral column

Q17 **Identify the following bones:**

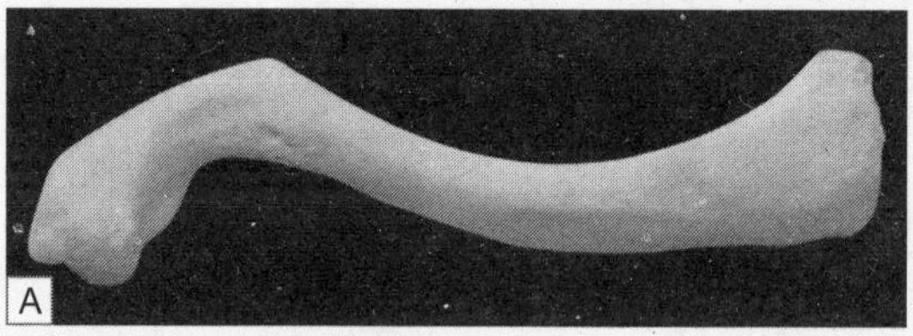

A. ______________________

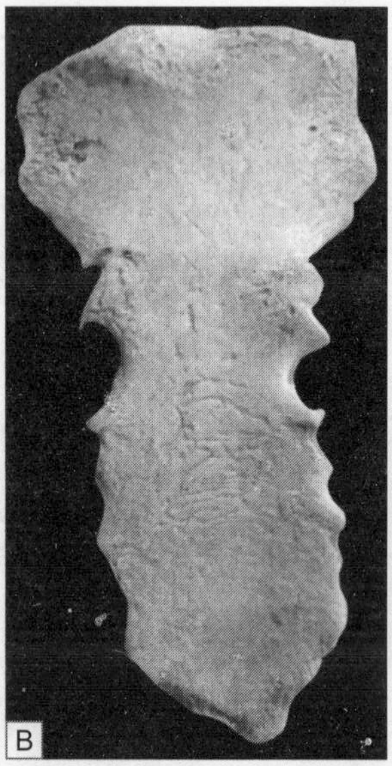

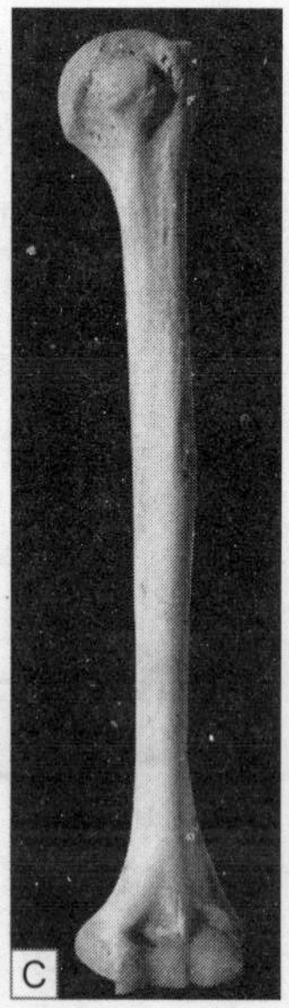

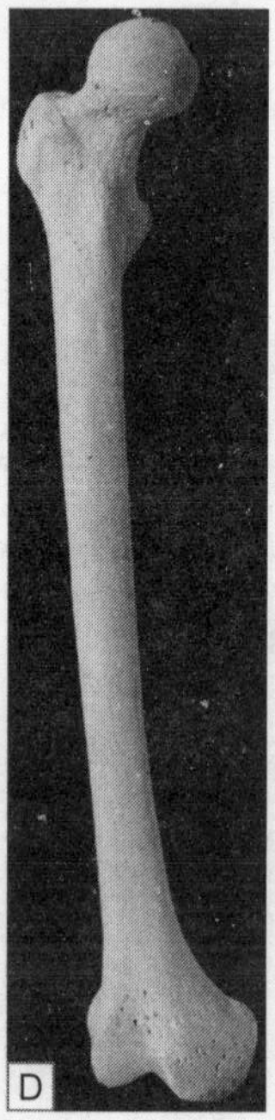

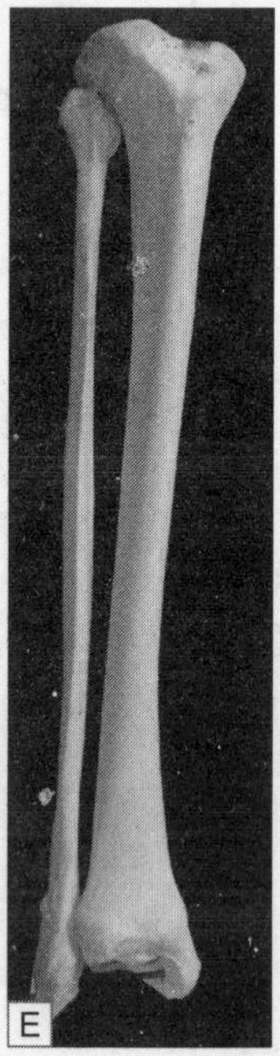

B. ______________________

C. ______________________

D. ______________________

E. ______________________

CHAPTER 8C

Musculoskeletal System—Joints

Q1 **Figure 8C.1 shows parts of a synovial joint. Identify the strucures**

A. ______________________________

B. ______________________________

C. ______________________________

D. ______________________________

E. ______________________________

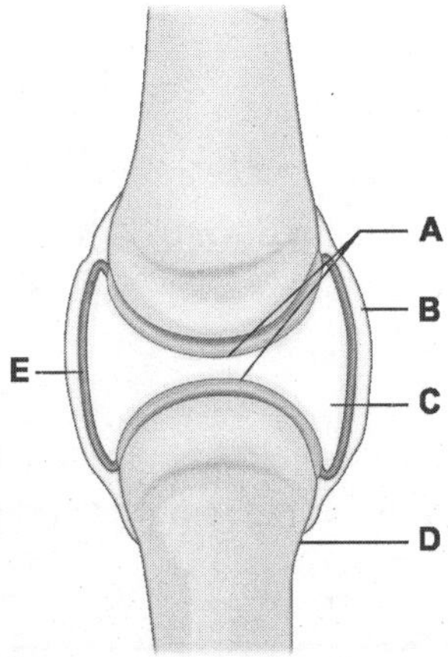

Fig. 8C.1

Q2 **Figure 8C.2 different types of synovial joints. Identify the type of joints.**

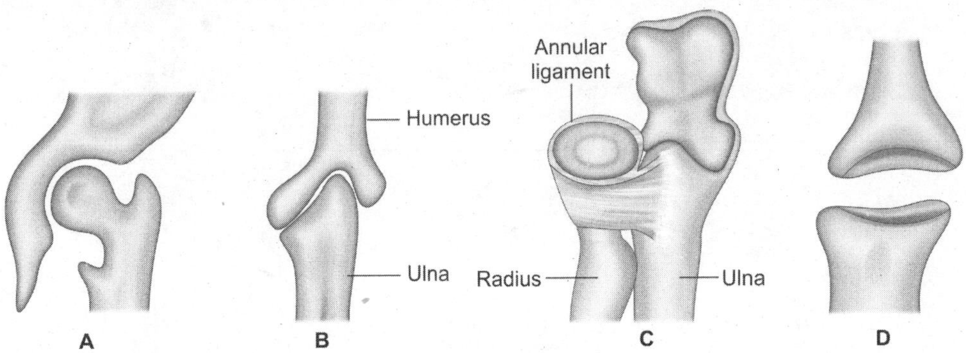

Fig. 8C.2

A. ______________________________

B. ______________________________

C. ______________________________

D. ______________________________

Q3 **Figure 8C.3 shows different movements possible at ankle joint. Identify the movements and name any 2 muscles which bring about that movement.**

A B

Fig. 8C.3

Movement

A. ______________________ B. ______________________

Muscles producing the movement

1. ______________________ 1. ______________________

2. ______________________ 2. ______________________

Q4 **Figure 8C.4 shows movements of thumb at first carpometacarpal joints. Identify the movements.**

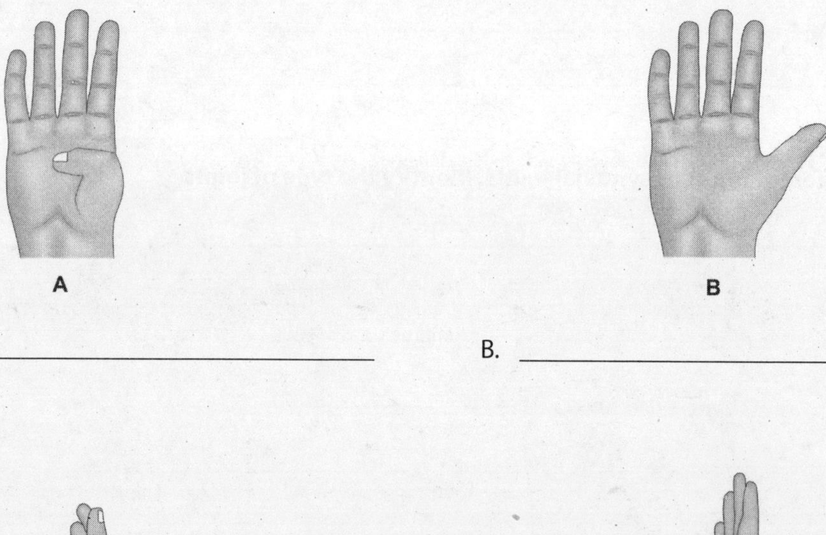

A B

A. ______________________ B. ______________________

C D

C. ______________________ D. ______________________

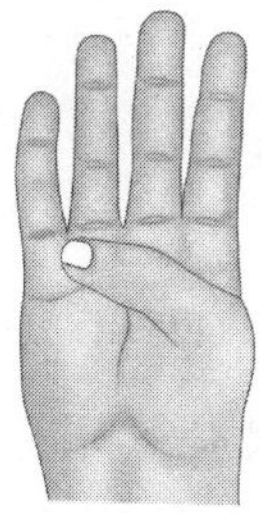

E

E. ______________________________

Fig. 8C.4

Q5 **Give a brief classification of joints.**

Q6 **Discuss in brief shoulder joint (type of joint, bones forming the joint, blood supply, nerve supply and movements). Draw a diagram to support the answer.**

Q7 Write short notes on

A. Synovial joints

B. Ball and socket joint

C. Hinge joint

D. Saddle joint

E. Carrying angle

F. Flexor retinaculum

E. Synovial fluid

Q8 **Match the following:**

	Joints of the body		Types of joints
A.	Joint between tooth and its socket	1.	Ball and socket joint
B.	Hip joint	2.	Condyloid or ellipsoid joint
C.	Elbow joint	3.	Gomphosis
D.	Atlantoaxial joint	4.	Hinge joint
E.	Wrist joint	5.	Pivotal joint

Q9 **Name the following:**

A. Joints of shoulder girdle

B. Muscles forming the rotator cuff

C. Bones forming the wrist joint

D. Bones forming the hip joint

E. Movements possible at knee joint

F. Structures passing under the cover of extensor retinaculum

____

____

G. Three varieities of fibrous joints

____

____

H. Name the muscles producing inversion and eversion of foot

____

____

Q10 True or False

A.	Joints between the skull bones are an example of fibrous joints	
B.	Joint between pubic symphysis is an example of cartilaginous joint	
C.	Nerves suplying the joint lie in its capsule	
D.	Pronation and supination of forearm takes place at inferior radioulnar joint	
E.	Knee joint is an example of compound joint	

CHAPTER

9 Respiratory System

Q1 **Figure 9.1 shows the respiratory passages. Identify the structures**

A. ____________________

B. ____________________

C. ____________________

D. ____________________

E. ____________________

F. ____________________

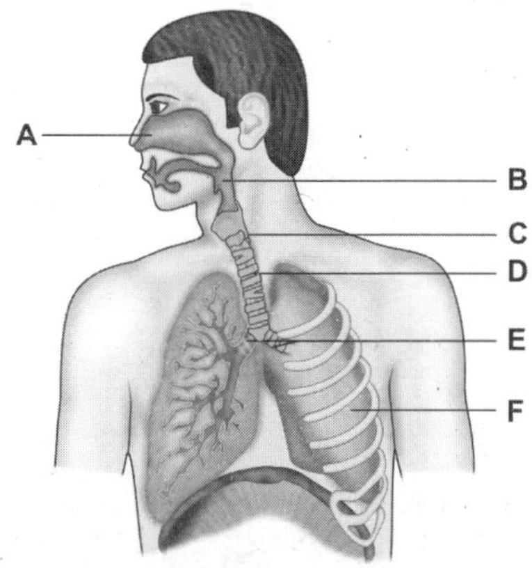

Fig. 9.1

Q2 **Figure 9.2 shows the anterior aspect of larynx. Identify the structures.**

A. ____________________

B. ____________________

C. ____________________

D. ____________________

E. ____________________

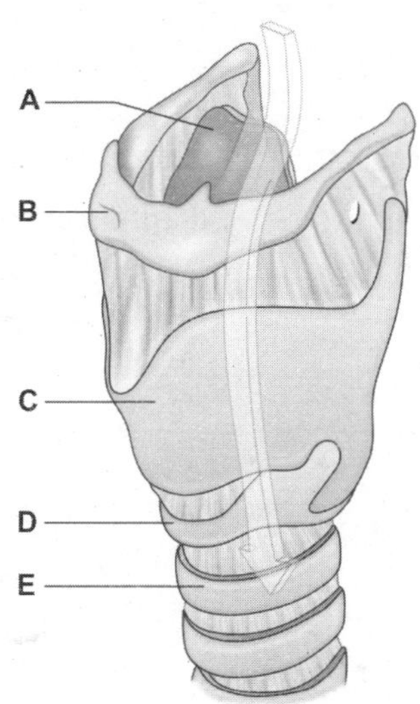

Fig. 9.2

Q3 **Figure 9.3 shows the tracheobronchial tree. Identify the structures.**

A. ______________________________

B. ______________________________

C. ______________________________

D. ______________________________

E. ______________________________

F. ______________________________

G. ______________________________

H. ______________________________

I. ______________________________

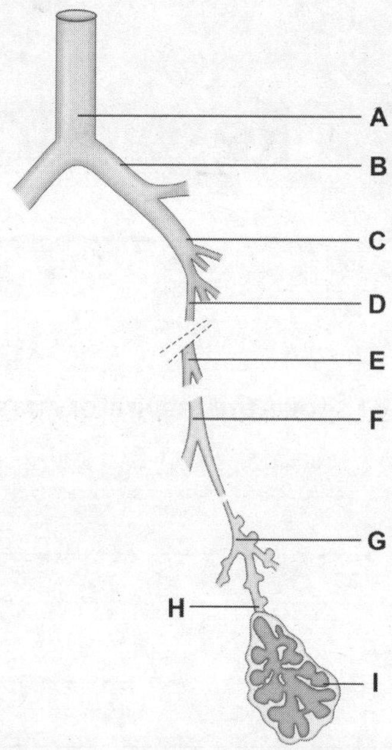

Fig. 9.3

Q4 **Draw a neatly labeled diagram to show arrangement of structures at the hilum of right lung.**

Q5 **Draw a neatly labeled diagram of spirogram showing various lung volumes and capacities.**

Q6 **Enumerate the functions of nose.**

Q7 **Enumerate the functions of larynx.**

Q8 **Enumerate the non-respiratory and defense functions of lungs.**

Q9 **Describe briefly how O_2 is transported from lungs to tissues.**

Q10 **Write short notes on:**

A. Paranasal air sinuses

B. Laryngeal cartilages

C. Bronchopulmonary segments

D. O_2-Hemoglobin dissociation curve

E. Hering Breuer reflex

F. Cyanosis

Q11 **Define the following terms**

A. Tidal volume

B. Vital capacity

C. Residual volume

D. Total lung capacity

E. Diffusing capacity

Q12 **Name the following:**

A. Structures present in the hilum of lungs from before backwards

B. Primary muscles of inspiration

C. Accessory muscles of inspiration

____

____

D. Adductors of vocal cord

____

____

E. Nerves supplying muscles of larynx

____

____

F. Lobes of right lung

____

____

G. Important lung volume with their average values

____

____

H. Paranasal air sinuses

____

____

I. Arteries forming the little's area.

____

____

J. Peripheral chemoreceptors

____

____

Q13 Write True (T) or False (F).

A.	Paranasal air sinuses open on nasal septum	
B.	Posterior nasal apertures are also called as choana.	
C.	Inferior concha is an independent bone.	
D.	Frontal sinus opens in middle meatus.	
E.	Paranasal air sinuses attain their full size at the time of birth.	
F.	Vocal cords are lined by stratified squamous epithelium	
G.	Vestibule refers to the external opening of the nose.	
H.	One molecule of hemoglobin can combine with 4 molecules of oxygen.	
I.	Carbon dioxide has less affinity for hemoglobin than oxygen.	
J.	The oxygen carrying capacity of 100 mL of blood is about 20 mL.	

Q14 **Match the following openings of sinuses with respective meatuses.**

	Sinuses		Meatus
A.	Nasolacrimal duct	1.	Superior meatus
B.	Maxillary sinus	2.	Inferior meatus
C.	Posterior ethmoidal sinus	3.	Middle meatus

Q15 **Match the following lung volumes/capacities with their respective average values.**

A.	Total lung capacity	1.	500 mL
B.	Vital capacity	2.	6 L
C.	Tidal volume	3.	1.2 L
D.	Residual volume	4.	4.8 L

CHAPTER 10A

Cardiovascular System—Heart

Q1 **Figure 10A.1 shows section of the heart. Identify the structure.**

A. ____________________

B. ____________________

C. ____________________

D. ____________________

E. ____________________

F. ____________________

G. ____________________

H. ____________________

I. ____________________

Identify the valves:

1. ____________________

2. ____________________

3. ____________________

4. ____________________

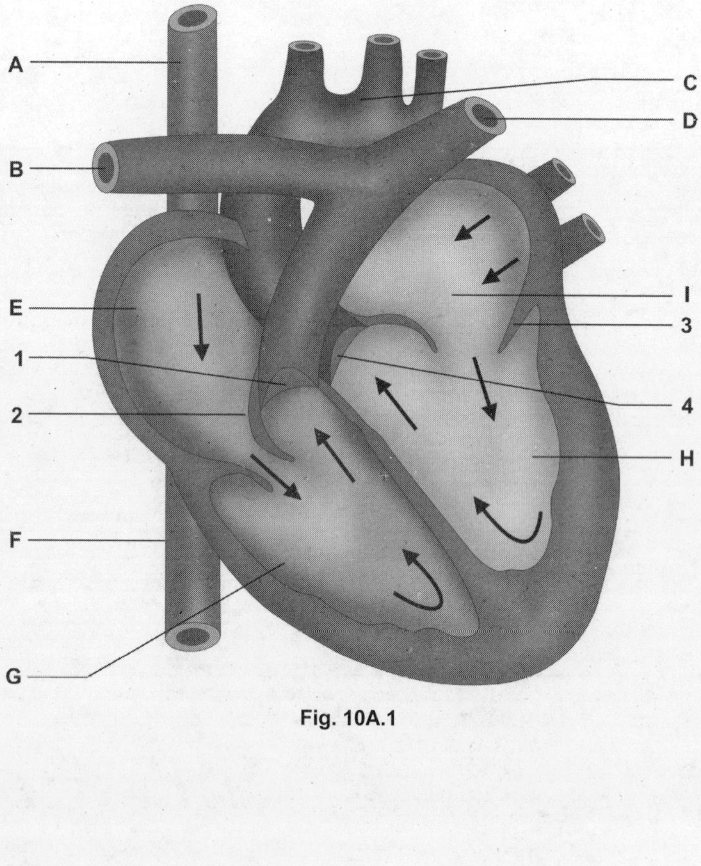

Fig. 10A.1

Q2 **Figure 10A.2 shows sternocostal surface of heart. Identify the following structures.**

A. ______________________

B. ______________________

C. ______________________

D. ______________________

E. ______________________

F. ______________________

G. ______________________

H. ______________________

I. ______________________

J. ______________________

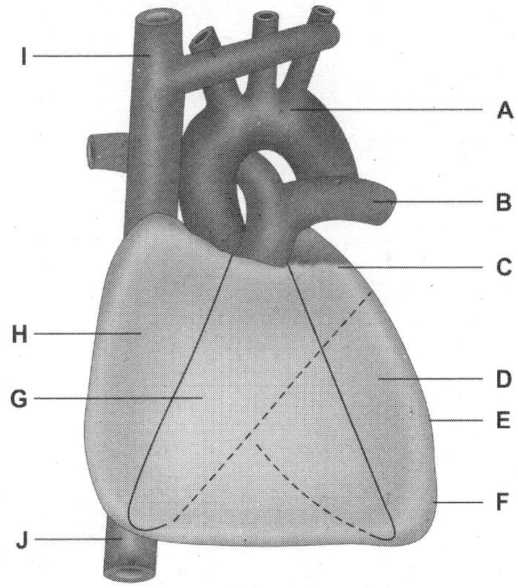

Fig. 10A.2

Q3 **Figure 10A.3 shows conducting of system of the heart. Identify the structures.**

A. ______________________

B. ______________________

C. ______________________

D. ______________________

E. ______________________

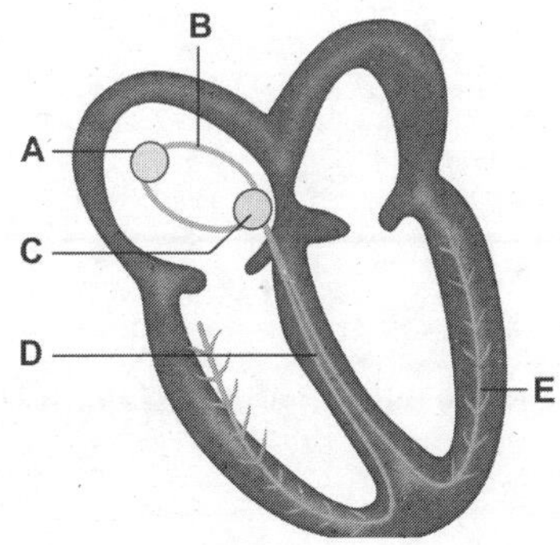

Fig. 10A.3

Q4 **Figure 10A.4 shows waves of normal ECG. Identify the waves. What do F, G and H indicate.**

A. ______________________

B. ______________________

C. ______________________

D. ______________________

E. ______________________

F. ______________________

G. ______________________

H. ______________________

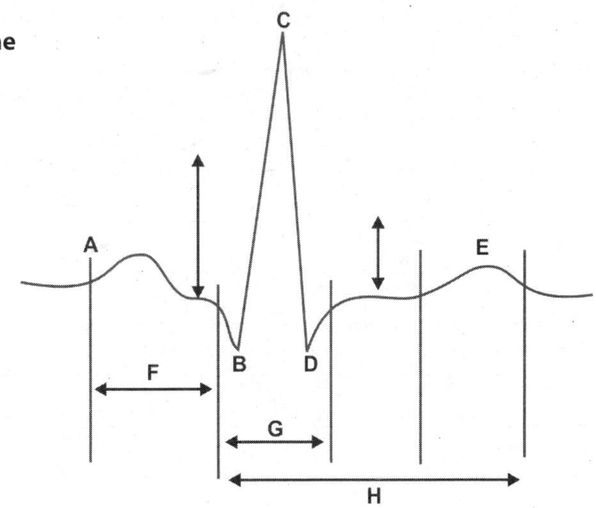

Fig. 10A.4

Q5 **Describe the structure and functions of heart.**

Q6 **Draw a flowchart to show connections between heart and various blood vessels.**

Q7 **Discuss briefly with the help of diagram pulmonary circulation.**

Q8 **Define the anatomical position of heart.**

Q9 **Discuss in brief the conducting system of the heart with a neatly labeled diagram.**

Q10 **Discuss in brief the effect of sympathetic stimulation on heart.**

Q11 **Write in briefly about the cardiac cycle.**

Q12 **Discuss briefly the regulation of blood pressure.**

Q13 **Define**

A. Cardiac output

B. Blood pressure and give its normal value in adult human

C. Mean arterial pressure

D. Electrocardiogram

E. Tachycardia

F. End-diastolic volume

G. Ejection fraction

Q14 **Write short notes on**

A. Factors affecting cardiac output

B. Coronary circulation

C. Role of renin–angiotensin in maintaining blood pressure

D. Heart sounds

E. Pulse

Q15 **Name the following:**

A. Layers of the wall of heart

B. The sulcus separating atria from ventricles

C. The point of maximum pulsation of heart

D. The pacemaker of the heart

E. The structure attaching papillary muscles to the cusp of tricuspid valve

F. Areas of heart supplied by right and left coronary artery, respectively

G. The largest vein of the heart

____

____

H. The three positive waves of JVP.

____

____

I. Valves of heart

____

____

Q16 Match the following parts of the heart with the main chambers contributing to its formation.

A.	Apex	1.	Right atrium
B.	Base	2.	Great vessels
C.	Right border	3.	Left ventricle
D.	Superior border	4.	Left atrium

Q17 Write True (T) or False (F)

A.	Cardiac muslce is involuntary	
B.	Atrioventricular node is the main pacemaker of the heart	
C.	Second heart sound is produced by closure of semilunar valves	
D.	Average heart rate in adult humans is 100/minute	
E.	Left ventricle contains 2 papillary muscles	

CHAPTER

10B Cardiovascular System—Blood Vessels

Q1 **Figure 10B.1 shows aorta and its parts and branches. Identify the following arteries.**

Parts of aorta

1. ______________________

2. ______________________

3. ______________________

4. ______________________

Branches

A. ______________________

B. ______________________

C. ______________________

D. ______________________

E. ______________________

F. ______________________

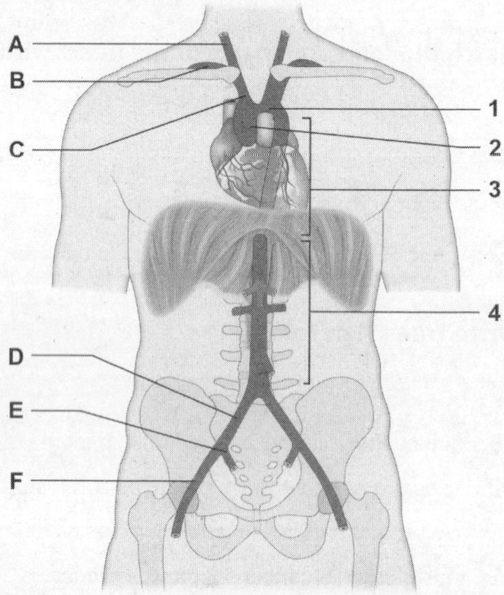

Fig. 10B.1

Q2 **Figure 10B.2 shows folds of dura mater and dural venous sinuses. Identify the folds and sinuses. Identify the structure H.**

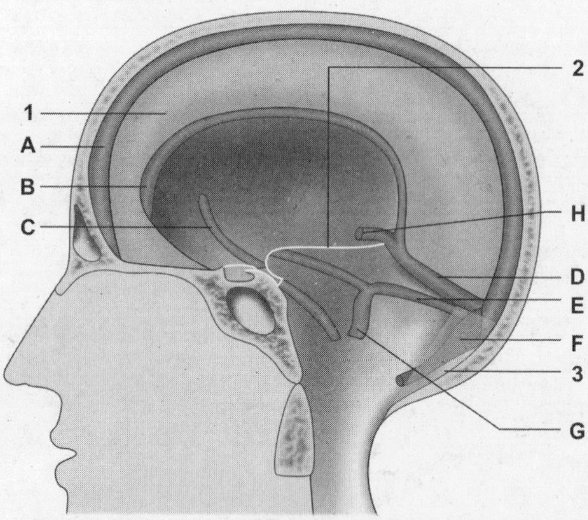

Fig. 10B.2

Folds

1. ______________________

2. ______________________

3. ______________________

Sinuses

A. ______________________

B. ______________________

C. ______________________

D. ______________________

E. ______________________

F. ______________________

G. ______________________

H. ______________________

Q3 **Figure 10B.3 shows arteries of upper limb. Identify the arteries.**

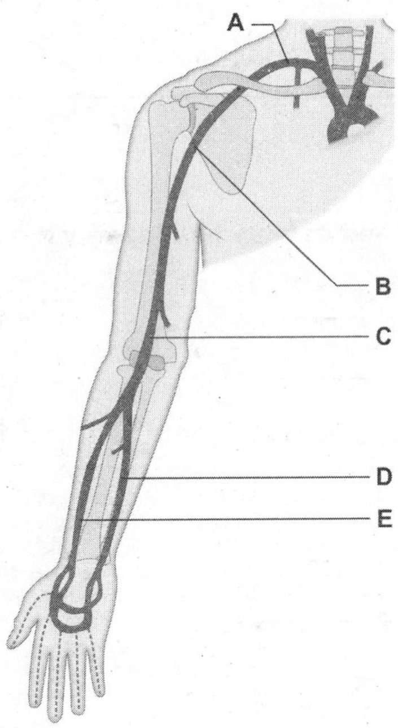

Fig. 10B.3

A. ______________________

B. ______________________

C. ______________________

D. ______________________

E. ______________________

Q4 **Figure 10B.4 shows veins of upper limb. Identify the veins.**

A. ____________________

B. ____________________

C. ____________________

D. ____________________

E. ____________________

F. ____________________

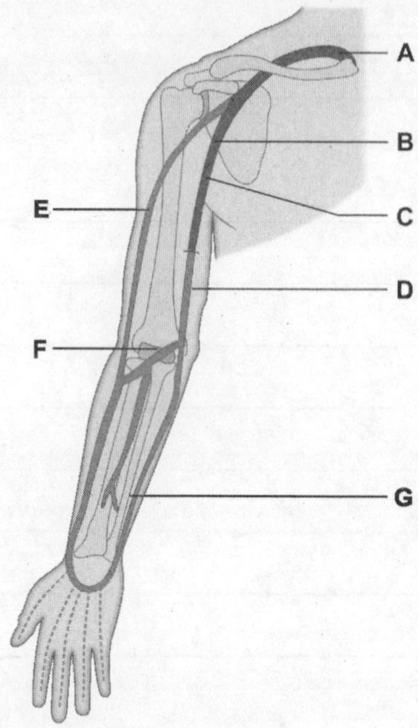

Fig. 10B.4

Q5 **Figure 10B.5 shows portal circulation and its branches. Identify the vessels.**

A. ____________________

B. ____________________

C. ____________________

D. ____________________

E. ____________________

F. ____________________

G. ____________________

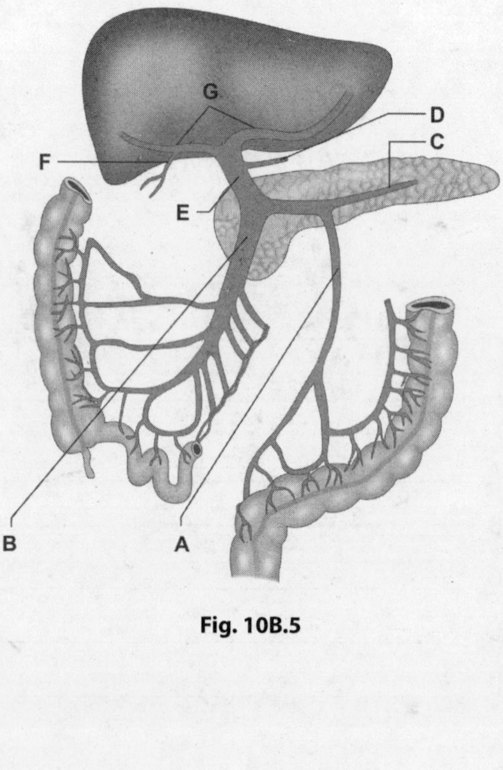

Fig. 10B.5

Q6 **Figure 10B.6 shows fetal circulation. Identify the structures.**

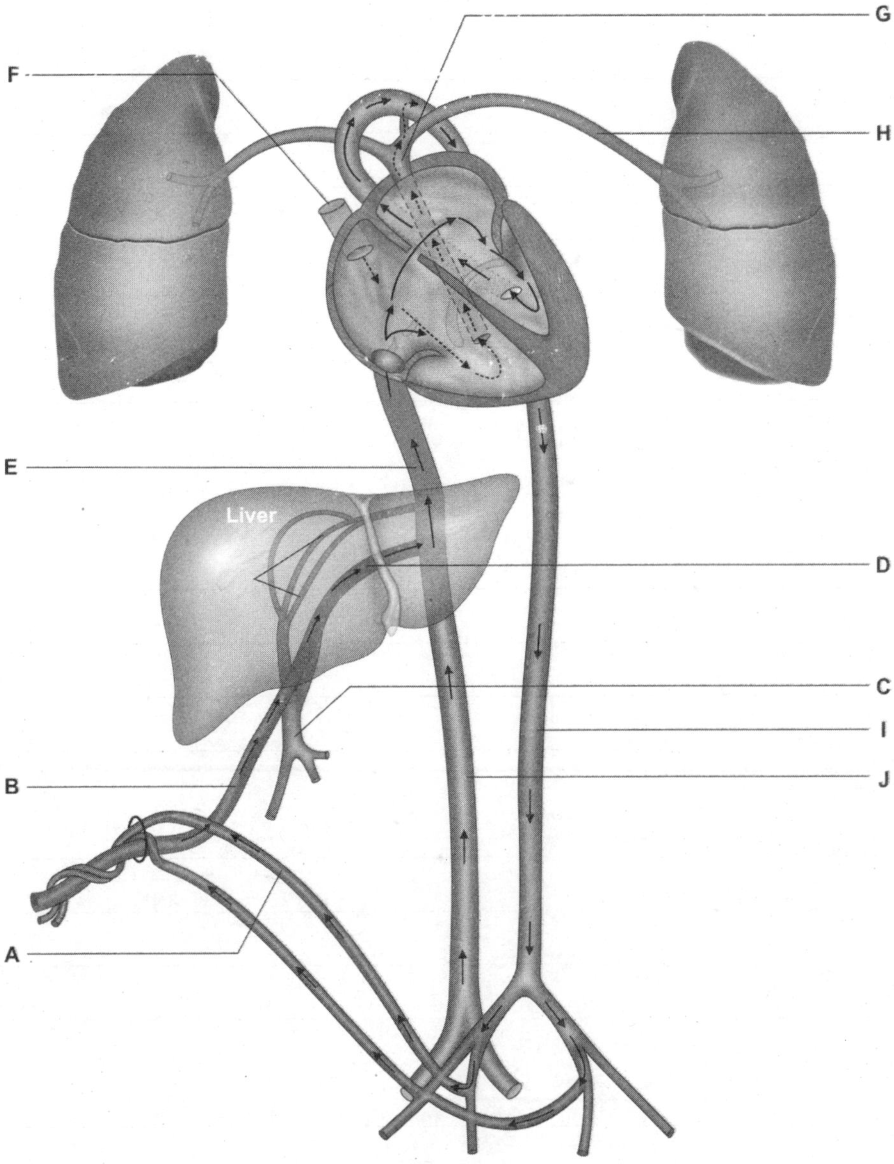

Fig. 10B.6

A. ______________________ F. ______________________

B. ______________________ G. ______________________

C. ______________________ H. ______________________

D. ______________________ I. ______________________

E. ______________________ J. ______________________

Q7 **Discuss briefly the fetal circulation.**

Q8 **Write short notes on:**

A. Elastic arteries

B. Portal circulation

C. Dural venous sinuses

D. Saphenous vein

Q9 **Enumerate:**

A. Three layers of arterial wall

B. Three main branches of arch of aorta

C. Branches of external carotid artery

D. Three unpaired branches of abdominal aorta

E. Veins forming the external jugular vein

F. Two terminal branches of brachial artery

G. Four superficial veins of upper limb

Q10 Name the following:

A. Vein formed by union of internal jugular vein and subclavian vein.

____

B. Main artery of upper limb.

____

C. Muscle dividing the axillary artery into three parts.

____

D. The main artery used for measuring arterial blood pressure.

____

E. The artery of foregut.

____

F. The largest vein in the body.

____

G. The artery which is a continuation of femoral artery.

____

H. The longest vein in the body.

____

Q11 Match the following fetal vessel with the remnants in adult.

A.	Umbilical vein	1.	Ligamentum arteriosum
B.	Umbilical artery	2.	Ligamentum venosum
C.	Ductus arteriosus	3.	Medial umbilical ligament
D.	Ductus venosus	4.	Ligamentum teres

Q12 Match the following

A.	Returns blood to heart from lower limbs	1.	Superior vena cava
B.	Returns blood to heart from head and upper body	2.	Inferior vena cava
C.	Chief artery of head and neck	3.	Superior mesenteric artery
D.	Vessel receiving the thoracic duct	4.	Common carotid artery
E.	Heart's blood system	5.	Left brachiocephalic vein
F.	Artery of midgut	6.	Coronary circulation

Q13 **Match the following arteries with their branches.**

	Artery		Branches
A.	Femoral artery	1.	Radial artery
B.	Popliteal artery	2.	Posterior intercostal artery
C.	Brachial artery	3.	Anterior circumflex humeral artery
D.	Axillary artery	4.	Inferior mesentric artery
E.	Abdominal aorta	5.	Profunda femoris artery
F.	Thoracic aorta	6.	Anterior tibial artery

Q14 **True or False:**

A.	The ascending aorta is the first part of aorta.	
B.	The right common carotid artery originates from the brachiocephalic trunk.	
C.	The middle meningeal artery is a branch of facial artery.	
D.	Internal carotid artery is a major contributor to circle of Willis which supplies the brain.	
E.	Subclavian artery continues as axillary artery.	
F.	Inferior mesenteric artery arises at the level of L1 vertebra.	
G.	Left ovarian vein/testicular vein drains into inferior vena cava.	
H.	Internal iliac artery is the principal artery of pelvic viscera.	
I.	Uterine artery is the branch of internal iliac artery.	
J.	Umbilical veins carry oxygenated blood from placenta to fetus.	

CHAPTER

11

Digestive System

Q1 **Figure 11.1 shows parts of digestive system. Identify the structures.**

A. ______________________

B. ______________________

C. ______________________

D. ______________________

E. ______________________

F. ______________________

G. ______________________

H. ______________________

I. ______________________

J. ______________________

K. ______________________

L. ______________________

M. ______________________

N. ______________________

O. ______________________

P. ______________________

Q. ______________________

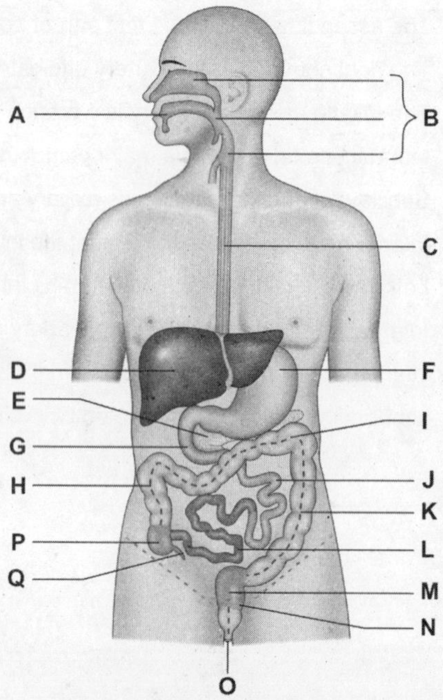

Fig. 11.1

Q2 **Figure 11.2 shows section though a tooth. Identify the structures.**

A. ______________________

B. ______________________

C. ______________________

D. ______________________

E. ______________________

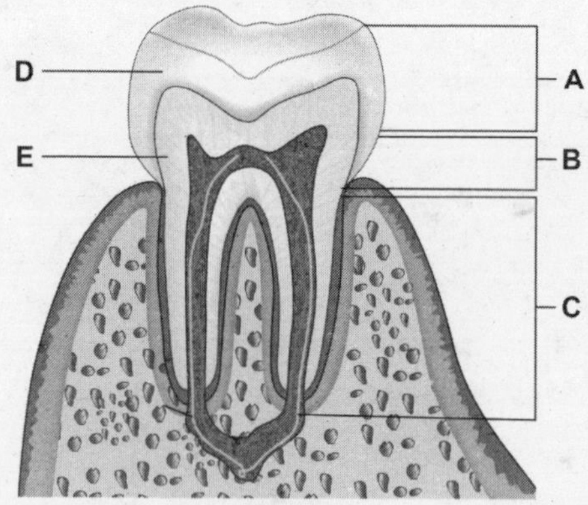

Fig. 11.2

Q3 **Draw a neatly labeled diagram of dorsal surface of tongue showing all the papillae, sulcus terminalis and foramen caecum.**

Q4 **Draw a neatly labeled diagram of stomach bed.**

Q5 **Figure 11.3 shows diagram of posterior surface of liver. Identify the lobes and ligaments. What structure is represented by E. What area is represented by F and what is its significance.**

Lobes:

A. ______________________

B. ______________________

C. ______________________

D. ______________________

E. ______________________

F. ______________________

Ligaments:

1. ______________________
2. ______________________
3. ______________________
4. ______________________

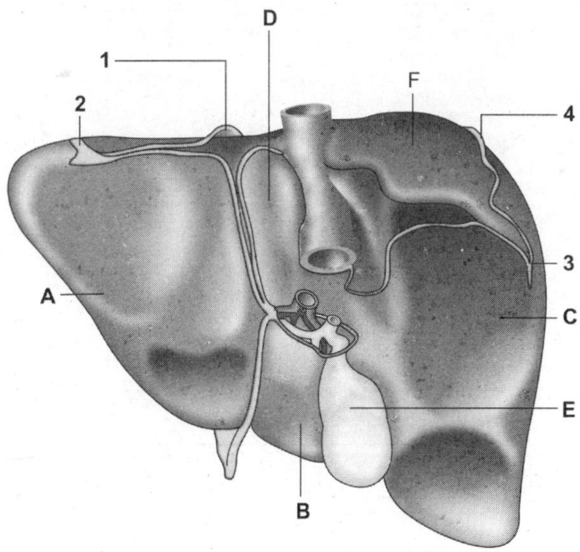

Fig. 11.3

Q6 **Draw flowchart showing composition of saliva**

Q7 **Draw flowchart showing composition of gastric juice.**

Q8 **Draw flowchart showing composition of bile**

Q9 **Write down the functions of**

A. Tongue

B. Liver

C. Stomach

D. Bile

E. Saliva

F. Tonsils

Q10 Write short notes on:

A. Tongue

B. Process of digestion

C. Waldeyer's ring

D. Salivary glands

E. Organs related to duodenum

F. Vermiform appendix

G. Organs associated with liver

H. Bile

I. Postprandial alkaline tide

Q11 **Tabulate the differences between:**

A. Tonsils and adenoids

Tonsils	Adenoids

B. Jejunum and ileum

Jejunum	Ileum

Q12 **Enlist the following**

A. Organs of digestive system

B. Parts of small intestine

C. Types of teeth

D. Types of papillae found on tongue

E. Three main sub divisions of pharynx

F. The three major salivary glands

G. The four main layers in the histology of gut wall

H. Any two GI hormones

I. Enzymes present in pancreatic juice

Q13 **Discuss briefly the structure of liver with the help of a diagram**

Q14 **Discuss briefly about gastric juice and phases of gastric secretion.**

Q15 **Name the following**

A. The cells of stomach secreting intrinsic factor for absorption of vit. B_{12}.

B. Duct formed by union of cystic duct and common hepatic duct.

C. Valve present in cystic duct

D. Primary bile acids

E. Duct formed by union of main pancreatic duct with accessory pancreatic duct.

Q16 **Define the following terms:**

A. Mastication

B. Deglutition

C. Chyme

D. Vomiting

E. Choleretics

____

____

Q17 **Match the following histological characteristics with the respective organ.**

A.	Circumvallate papillae	1.	Parotid gland
B.	Serous acini`	2.	Stomach
C.	Chief cells	3.	Pancreas
D.	Crypts of Leiberkuhn	4.	Tongue
E.	Taenia coli	5.	Intestine
F.	Portal triad	6.	Colon
G.	Islets of Langerhans	7.	Liver

Q18 **Match the following digestive organs with their blood supply.**

A.	Tongue	1.	Gastric artery
B.	Pharynx	2.	Lingual artery
C.	Stomach	3.	Portal vein
D.	Duodenum	4.	Ascending pharyngeal artery
E.	Liver	5.	Pancreaticoduodenal artery

Q19 **Match the following glands with their respective ducts.**

A.	Pancreas	1.	Whartons duct
B.	Parotid	2.	Cystic duct
C.	Submaxillary	3.	Duct of Wirsung and Santorini
D.	Gall bladder	4.	Stensen duct

Q20 **Write True (T) or False (F)**

A.	Palate separates oropharynx from the oral cavity	
B.	Tongue is covered by stratified squamous epithelium	
C.	Nasopharynx is lined by ciliated columnar epithelium	
D.	Submandibular gland is an example of mixed serous and mucous gland.	
E.	Lower esophageal sphincter has a pressure of 5-10 mm of Hg.	
F.	Pyloric antrum open into the duodenum	
G.	Lesser curvature gives attachment to lesser omentum	
H.	Duodenum is a retroperitoneal organ	
I.	Hepatopancreatic ampulla of Vater opens into the second part of duodenum	
J.	Achalasia is a condition in which there is a decreased tone of lower esophageal sphincter	

CHAPTER

12

Urinary System

Q1 **Figure 12.1 shows parts of urinary system. Identify the structures.**

A. ______________________________

B. ______________________________

C. ______________________________

D. ______________________________

E. ______________________________

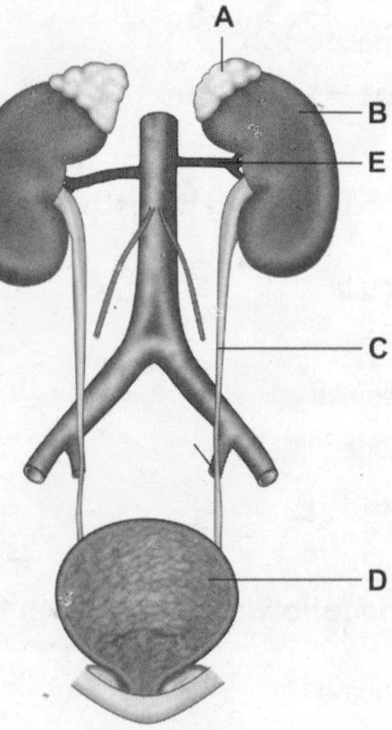

Fig. 12.1

Q2 **Figure 12.2 shows structure of kidney. Identify the structures.**

A. ______________________________

B. ______________________________

C. ______________________________

D. ______________________________

E. ______________________________

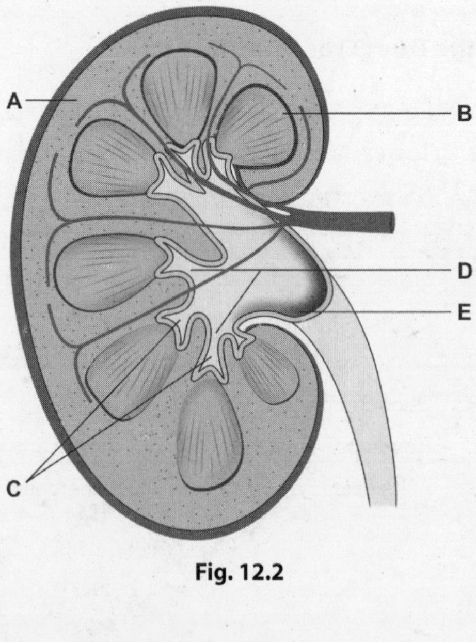

Fig. 12.2

Q3 **Figure 12.3 shows parts of a nephron. Identify the structures.**

(i) A. ____________________

B. ____________________

C. ____________________

D. ____________________

E. ____________________

F. ____________________

G. ____________________

H. ____________________

(ii) In the figure draw a line to demarcate parts of nephron seen in cortex and seen in medulla.

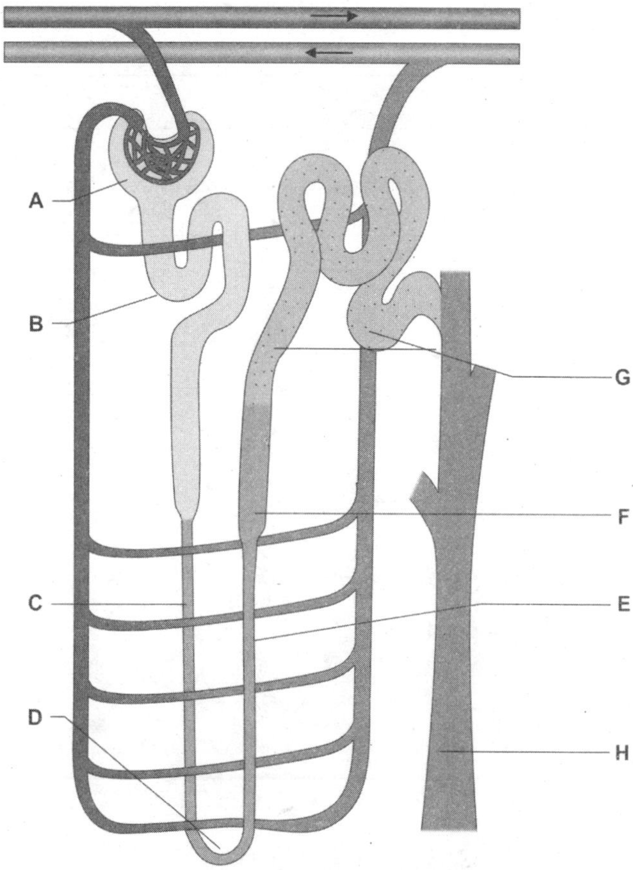

Fig. 12.3

Q4 **Discuss briefly the functions of kidney.**

____

____

____

____

____

____

Q5 **Describe the structure of nephron along with a diagram.**

____

____

____

Q6 **Draw flowcharts to show**

A. Passage of urine

B. Passage of blood through kidney

C. Composition of urine

Q7 **Draw a neatly labelled diagram to show**

A. Glomerular capsule

B. Juxtaglomerular appratus

C. Glomerular filtration membrane

D. Draw and label the structures related posteriorly to the right kidney.

Q8

Enlist

A. The three major processes involved in urine formation.

____

____

____

B. The structures seen at the hilum of the kidney from anterior to posterior.

____

____

____

C. The parts of a nephron.

____

____

____

D. The structures forming the glomerular filtration membrane.

____

____

____

E. Structures forming the juxtaglomerular apparatus.

Q9 **Write short notes on:**

A. Physiology of urine formation

B. Role of ADH in concentration of urine

C. Tubular reabsorption

D. Tubular secretion

E. Renin angiotensin system

____

____

____

____

____

Q10 **Define**

A. Glomerular filtration rate

____

____

____

B. Mictuirition

____

____

____

C. Transport maximum

____

____

____

D. Renal threshold

____

____

____

Q11 **Match the following:**

	Part of nephron		Function
A.	Glomerular capsule	1.	Selective reabsorption of ions like Na^+ and HCO_3^- and secretion of H^+ ions
B.	Proximal convoluted tubule	2.	Final concentration of urine
C.	Distal convoluted tubule	3.	Filtration of molecules and water from blood
D.	Collecting duct	4.	Selective reabsorption of glucose and water

Q12 Name the following:

A.	The part where maximum reabsorption occurs.	
B.	The substances not filtered through glomerulus.	
C.	Hormone produced by atrial muscles which increases excretion of sodium	
D.	The involuntary sphincter of urethra	
E.	The hormone which increases water reabsorption in DCT and CT	

Q13 Write True (T) or False (F).

A.	Blood is carried out of the glomerulus by the efferent arteriole	
B.	Angiotensin II increases sodium reabsorption in proximal tubule	
C.	At the time of micturition, detrussor muscle relaxes	
D.	Angiotensin converting enzyme (ACE) is secreted from proximal convoluted tubule	
E.	90% of blood to the kidney flows to the cortical region and 10% to medulla	

CHAPTER

13 Introduction to Genetics

Q1 **Figure 13.1 shows structure of a chromosome. Identify the parts.**

A. ______________________________

B. ______________________________

C. ______________________________

D. ______________________________

E. ______________________________

F. ______________________________

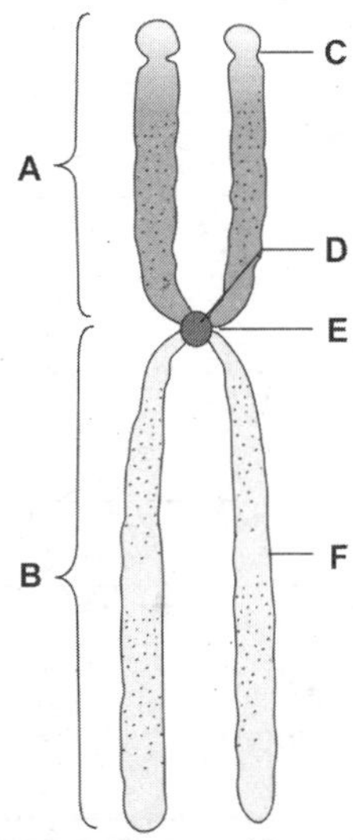

Fig. 13.1

Q2 **Figure 13.2 shows different types of chromosomes. Identify them.**

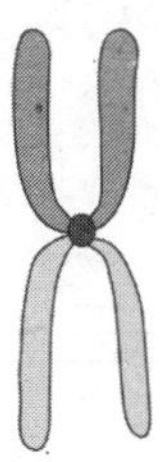

A. ______________________________

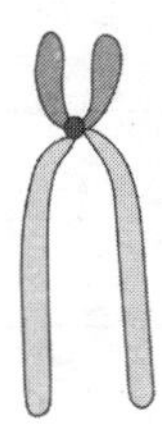

B. ______________________________

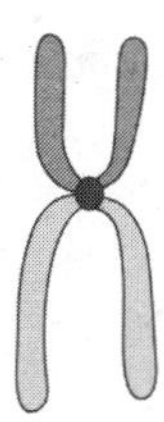

C. ______________________________

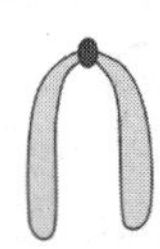

D. ______________________________

Q3

Discuss briefly the basic structure of DNA and draw a diagram.

Q4

Define

A. Diploid cell

B. Karyotype

C. Cytogenetics

D. Genetic code

E. Acrocentric chromosome

F. Nucleotide

Q5 **Write short notes on**

A. Mitosis

B. Dominant inheritance

C. X-linked inheritance

Q6 **Give two examples of disorders with autosomal recessive inheritance.**

Q7 **What is karyotype of**

A. Normal female

B. Normal male

C. Down's syndrome

D. Turner's syndrome

____

____

Q8 What is Barr body? How many Barr bodies are present in patients of Klinefelter's syndrome?

____

____

____

____

____

____

____

Q9 True or False

1.	There are 22 pairs of autosomes in humans	
2.	If a sperm containing Y chromosome fertilizes an ovum, the zygote will be a genetic female with chromosomal pattern 44 + XY	
3.	The double helix model of DNA was proposed by James Watson and Harry Crick	
4.	Genetic information is stored in the DNA molecule in the form of triplet code	
5.	Adenine on one strand of DNA is always linked to guanine on the other strand	
6.	DNA plays a vital role in the synthesis of proteins	
7.	The chromosome number is reduced to half in meiosis II	
8.	Monosomy refers to a condition in which chromosome number is reduced to half	
9.	Gametes are an example of haploid cells	
10.	The stage of a cell in between division is called interphase	

CHAPTER

14 Reproductive System

FEMALE REPRODUCTIVE SYSTEM

Q1 **Figure 14.1 shows internal organs of female reproductive system. Identify the structures. Parts of fallopian tubes are shown by 1 to 4. Identify the parts. What structure does X represents in the figure.**

A. ______________________

B. ______________________

C. ______________________

D. ______________________

E. ______________________

F. ______________________

G. ______________________

X. ______________________

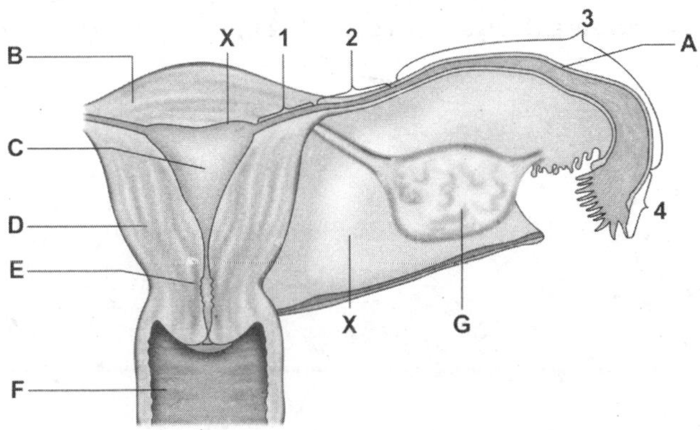

Fig. 14.1

Parts of fallopian tube

1. ______________________
2. ______________________
3. ______________________
4. ______________________

Q2 **Figure 14.2 shows parts of uterus. Label the following parts.**

A. Fundus

B. Body

C. Isthmus

D. Cervix

E. Internal Os

F. External Os

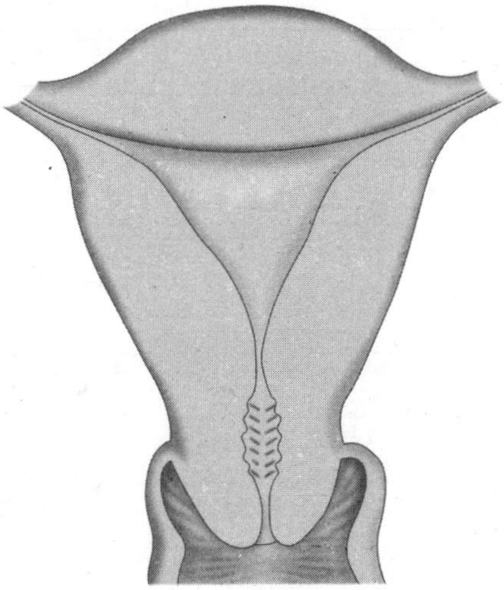

Fig. 14.2

Q3 **Draw a diagram to show supports of uterus.**

Q4 **Draw a flowchart to show the process of oogenesis.**

Q5 **Write down the functions of:**

A. Fallopian tubes

B. Ovaries

Q6 **Discuss briefly the menstrual cycle. Support your answer with suitable diagrams.**

Q7 **Discuss briefly mammary glands. Supports your answer with suitable diagrams.**

Q8

Name the following:

A. Three layers of uterus

B. The part which makes the junction between body of uterus and cervix

C. The place where cervix opens into the vagina

D. Female gonad

E. Epithelium lining the vaginal part of cervix

F. Normal position of uterus in a female

G. Three layers of endometrium seen during proliterative phase

Q9

Define the following:

A. Puberty

B. Menopause

C. Menarche

D. Caruncularae myrtiformes

Q10 **Write short notes:**

A. Bartholin's glands

B. Supports of uterus

C. Pelvic diaphragm

D. Perineal body

E. Graafian follicle

Q11 **Write True (T) or False (F):**

A.	Labia minora are covered with hair and their inner surface has large sebaceous glands.	
B.	External os is pin point/circular in nulliparous females.	
C.	Cervix is covered by peritoneum on all sides.	
D.	Under the influence of progesterone, cervical mucus becomes thick and tenacious.	
E.	Montgomery's tubercles are enlarged sweat glands.	
F.	Uterus and fallopian tube develop from Wolffian duct (mesonephric ducts)	

Q12 **Match the following:**

	Part of female reproductive system		Lining
A.	Endometrium	1.	Stratified squamous epithelium
B.	Vagina	2.	Transitional epithelium
C.	Fallopian tubes	3.	Columnar epithelium
D.	Female urethra	4.	Ciliated columnar epithelium

Q13 **Match the following parts of female genital system homologus with the male genital system.**

A.	Ovaries	1.	Penis
B.	Labia majora	2.	Testes
C.	Clitoris	3.	Scrotum
D.	Bartholin's gland	4.	Bulb of penis
E.	Bulb of vestibule	5.	Cowper's glands

Q14 **Match the following:**

	Female genital organs		Lymphatic drainage
A.	Vulva	1.	External and internal iliac nodes
B.	Uterus	2.	Superficial inguinal nodes
C.	Ovary	3.	Axillary nodes
D.	Breast	4.	Lateral aortic (Paraaortic)

Q15

Match the following

A.	FSH	1.	Secreted by ovary in follicular phase
B.	LH	2.	Secreted by corpus luteum
C.	Estrogen	3.	Responsible for growth of follicles
D.	Progesterone	4.	Responsible for ovulation

Q16

Choose the correct answer.

A. In a 40 day menstrual cycle, ovulation occurs at ________________ (14th day/26th day)

B. Corpus luteum secretes ________________ (progesterone/FSH)

C. Ovulation occurs due to ________________ (LH surge/FSH surge)

D. Completion of second meiotic division results in expulsion of ________________ (first polar body/second polar body)

E. Karyotype of secondary oocytes is ________________ (23X/46XX)

F. Appearance of first menstrual period is ________________ (menopause/menarche)

G. Ligament which keep the uterus in anteverted position ________________ (round ligament/broad ligament)

H. Chief hormone of secretory phase is ________________ (estrogen/progesterone)

MALE REPRODUCTIVE SYSTEM

Q1 **Figure 14.3 shows parts of male reproductive system. Identify the parts.**

A. ______________________

B. ______________________

C. ______________________

D. ______________________

E. ______________________

F. ______________________

G. ______________________

H. ______________________

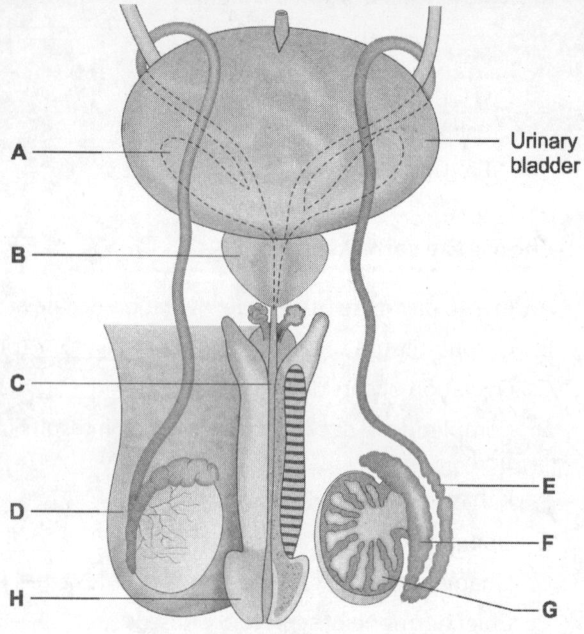

Fig. 14.3

Q2 **Draw a flowchart showing steps of spermatogenesis.**

Q3 **Figure 14.4 shows the structure of a spermatozoan. Label the regions marked by A, B and C and identify the parts marked by 1 to 5.**

Parts

1. ______________________
2. ______________________
3. ______________________
4. ______________________
5. ______________________

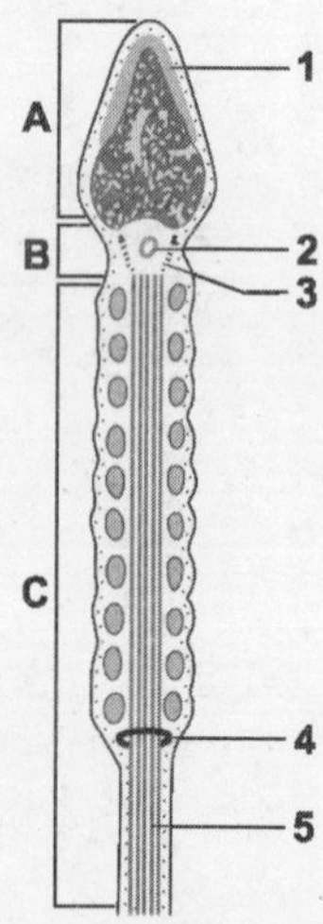

Fig. 14.4

Regions

A. ______________________________

B. ______________________________

C. ______________________________

Q4

Name:

A. External genital organs of male

____

____

____

B. Internal genital organs of male

____

____

____

C. Structure which suspends testes in the scrotum

____

____

____

D. Covering of testes

____

____

____

E. Comma-shaped structure situated along the posterior border of the testes.

____

____

____

F. Structure which transmits spermatozoa from epididymis to ejaculatory duct.

____

____

____

Q5 **Short Notes:**

A. Prostrate gland

B. Functions of testes

C. Structure of sperm

D. Pubertal change in males

Q6 **Write True (T) or False (F).**

A.	Normal pH of semen is 7.5.	
B.	After ejaculation sperms can survive for 5-6 days.	
C.	LH is the main hormone promoting testosterone secretion from testes.	
D.	Vasectomy refers to cutting of seminal vesicles	
E.	Maturation of sperms takes place in epididymis	
F.	Right testicular vein drains into inferior vena cava	
G.	In the fetus, the testes develop in the lumbar region and descends later on to reach bottom of scrotum by ninth month	
H.	The duct of seminal vesicles joins vas deferens to form the ejaculatory duct	

CHAPTER

15

Endocrine System

Q1 **Figure 15.1 shows endocrine glands in the body. Identify the following.**

A. ______________________

B. ______________________

C. ______________________

D. ______________________

E. ______________________

F. ______________________

G. ______________________

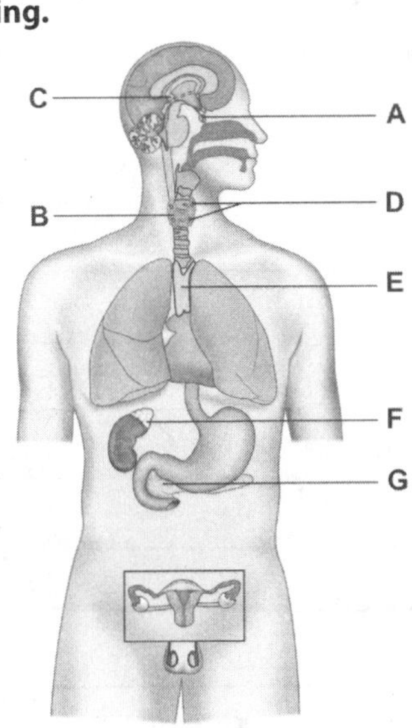

Fig. 15.1

Q2 **Give a brief classification of hormones on the basis of their chemical nature.**

____

____

____

____

____

____

Q3 **Give functions/actions of the following hormones:**

A. FSH

____

____

____

B. Prolectin

C. Growth hormone

D. Thyroid hormone

E. Calcitonin

F. Aldosterone

G. Glucocorticoids

H. Insulin

Q4 **Discuss briefly the process of formation and secretion of thyroid hormone.**

Q5 **Write short notes on:**

A. Regulation of secretion of hormones

B. Hypothalamohypophyseal portal system

C. Regulation of calcium metabolism

D. Milk ejection reflex

Q6 Enlist:

A. Hormones secreted by anterior pituitary

B. Hormones secreted by posterior pituitary

C. Hormones of thyroid gland

D. Hormones associated with calcium metabolism.

E. Subdivisions of pituitary gland

F. Hormones of adrenal medulla

Q7 Name the following:

A. The gland referred to as 'master endocrine gland'

B. The tract connecting posterior lobe of pituitary gland with hypothalamus

____

C. Arteries supplying the pituitary gland

____

D. Hormone released by pituitary which stimulates the release of thyroid hormone

____

E. Hormone which stimulates milk secretion during pregnancy

____

F. Hormones which results in ejection of milk.

____

G. Hormone secreted by posterior pituitary which acts on collecting duct of kidney and increases water reabsorption

____

H. Cell secreting calcitonin

____

I. Organ that acts as a reservoir for calcium

____

J. Hormone which increases blood calcium levels by bone resorption

____

K. Part of adrenal gland secreting mineralocorticoids

____

L. Disease that occurs due to excess cortisol production

____

Q8 **Match the following hormones with their action**

	Hormone		Actions
A.	Thyroid	1.	Increases serum calcium levels
B.	Calcitonin	2.	Causes uterine contractions
C.	Parathormone	3.	Increases basal metabolic rate
D.	Oxytocin	4.	Utilization of glucose
E.	Insulin	5.	Lowers serum calcium levels
F.	Glucagon	6.	Increased blood levels of glucose

Q9 Write True (T) or False (F):

A.	Optic chiasma is intimately related to pituitary gland	
B.	Melanocyte stimulating hormone (MSH) is secreted by pars intermedia of pituitary	
C.	Growth hormone acts via somatomedins	
D.	Antidiuretic hormone is an example of steroid hormone	
E.	The false capsule of thyroid gland is formed by pretracheal layer of deep cervical fascia	
F.	Superior thyroid arteries arise from first part of subclavian artery	
G.	Majority of T_3 and T_4 in blood are bound to plasma proteins	
H.	In hyperthyroidism, levels of TSH are increased	
I.	Insulin is secreted by β-cells of pancreas	
J.	Liver is the principal target organ of hormone glucagon	

CHAPTER 16

Special Senses

Q1 **Figure 16.1 shows parts of the ear. Identify the structures**

A. ________________________________

B. ________________________________

C. ________________________________

D. ________________________________

E. ________________________________

F. ________________________________

G. ________________________________

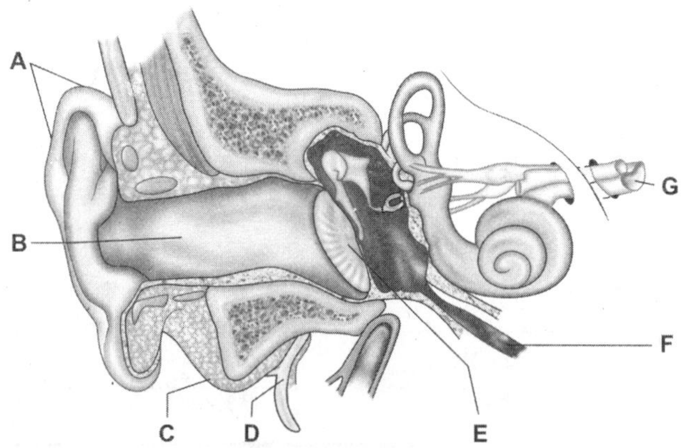

Fig. 16.1

Q2 **Figure 16.2 shows parts of middle ear as skin in coronal section. Identify the structures. What do area 'X' and 'Y' represents.**

A. ________________________________

B. ________________________________

C. ________________________________

D. ________________________________

E. ________________________________

X. ________________________________

Y. ________________________________

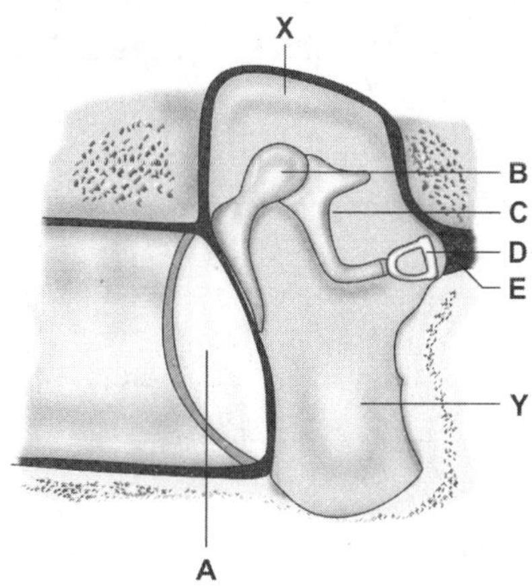

Fig. 16.2

Q3 **Figure 16.3 shows structure of cochlear canal. Identify the structures.**

A. ____________________

B. ____________________

C. ____________________

D. ____________________

E. ____________________

F. ____________________

G. ____________________

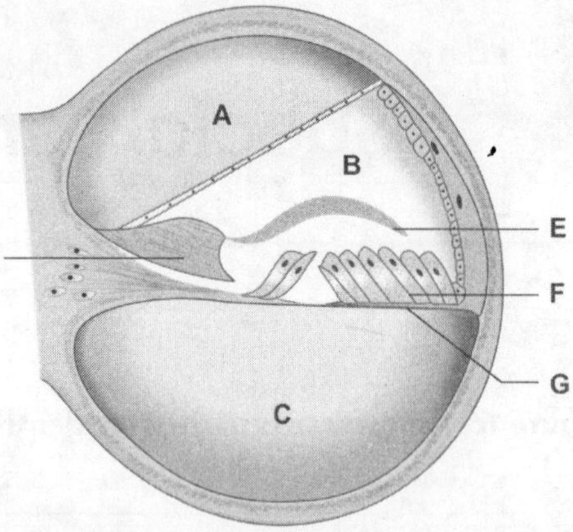

Fig. 16.3

Q4 **Figure 16.4 shows perilymphatic and endolymphatic systems of cochlea. Identify areas A, B and C. Name the fluids found in each of these areas. What do areas 'X', 'Y' and 'Z' represent? Write the clinical significance of 'Z'**

A. ____________________

B. ____________________

C. ____________________

X. ____________________

Y. ____________________

Z. ____________________

Fluids in A. ____________________

B. ____________________

C. ____________________

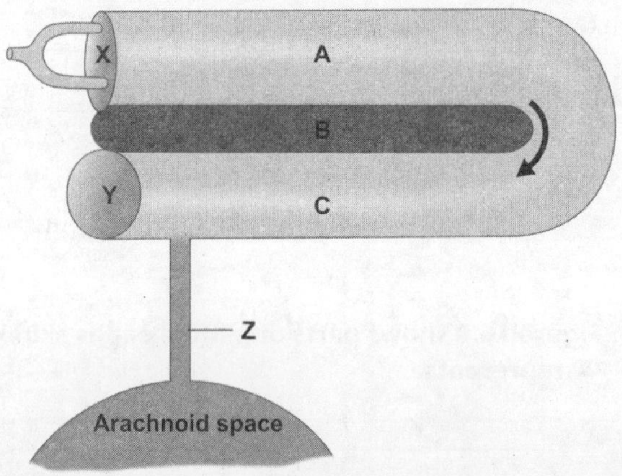

Fig. 16.4

Q5 **Figure 16.5 shows lacrimal apparatus. Identify the structures.**

A. ____________________

B. ____________________

C. ____________________

D. ____________________

E. ____________________

F. ____________________

G. ____________________

H. ____________________

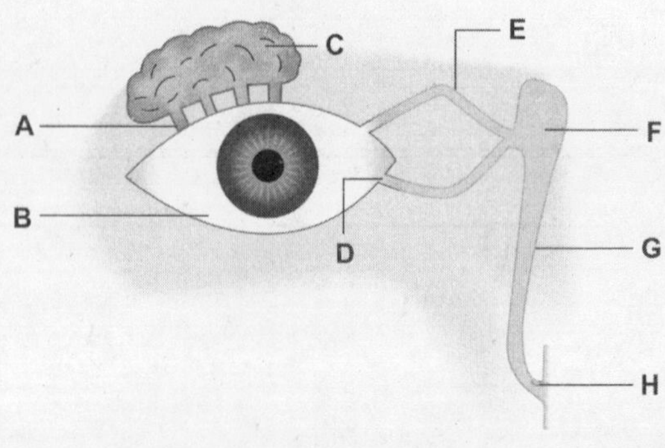

Fig. 16.5

Q6 **Figure 16.6 shows structure of eyeball. Identify the structures.**

A. ______________________

B. ______________________

C. ______________________

D. ______________________

E. ______________________

F. ______________________

G. ______________________

H. ______________________

I. ______________________

J. ______________________

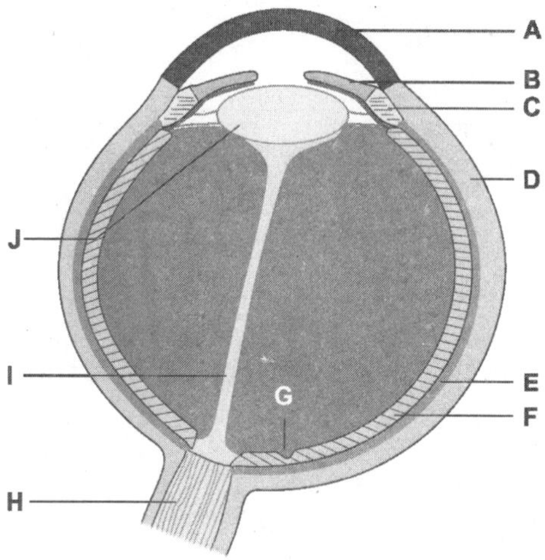

Fig. 16.6

Q7 **Draw a neatly labeled diagram of**

A. Structure of tympanic membrane

B. Auditory pathway

C. Taste pathway

D. Papillary light reflex

Q8 **Figure 16.7 shows visual pathway. Identify the parts.**

A. ______________________

B. ______________________

C. ______________________

D. ______________________

E. ______________________

F. ______________________

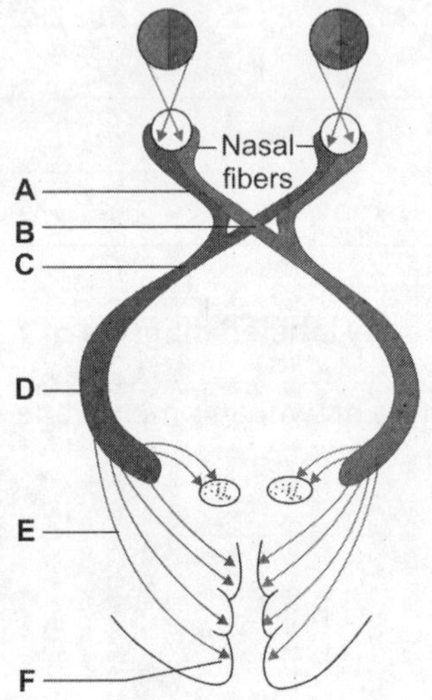

Fig. 16.7

Q9 **Discuss briefly the effect of lesions in visual pathway.**

Q10 Write Short notes an

A. Inner ear fluids

B. Organ of Corti

C. Physiology of hearing

D. Binocular and monocular vision

E. Accomodation reflex

Q11 **Enlist:**

A. Three main parts of ear.

B. Three ear ossicles.

C. Recti muscles of the eye.

D. Layers of eyeball and structures constituting the layers.

E. Functions of sclera.

F. The fluid present in the eye.

G. Photoreceptors in the retina

Q12 **Match the following muscles of the eye with their nerve supply.**

A.	Lateral rectus	1.	Oculomotor nerve
B.	Superior oblique	2.	Abducent nerve
C.	Superior rectus	3.	Trochlear nerve

Q13 **Choose the correct answer.**

A. The end organs for the sense of taste are called ________________ (taste bud/taste bulb)

B. Auricle consists of a thin plate of ________________ (fibrous cartilage/elastic cartilage)

C. Tympanic membrane shows a central depression called ________________ (umbo/macula lutea)

D. The floor of middle ear is related to ________________ (internal jugular vein/internal carotid artery)

E. The site of maximum acuity of vision in retina ________________ (ciliary body/fovea centralis)

Q14 **Write True (T) or False (F).**

A.	There are five basic tastes	
B.	Tympanic membrane forms a partition between external ear and inner ear	
C.	The lateral one-third of auditory tube is cartilaginous	
D.	Cochlea makes two and a half turns around modiolus	
E.	Fovea centralis contains cone only	

CHAPTER

17

Skin and Temperature Regulation

Q1 **Figure 17.1 shows skin & its related structures. Identify the layers A, B and structures C, D, E.**

A. ____________________

B. ____________________

C. ____________________

D. ____________________

E. ____________________

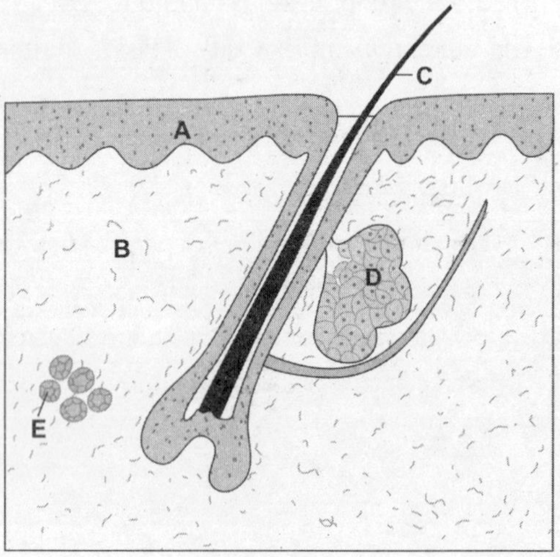

Fig. 17.1

Q2 **Figure 17.2 shows layers of skin. Identify the layers.**

A. ____________________

B. ____________________

C. ____________________

D. ____________________

E. ____________________

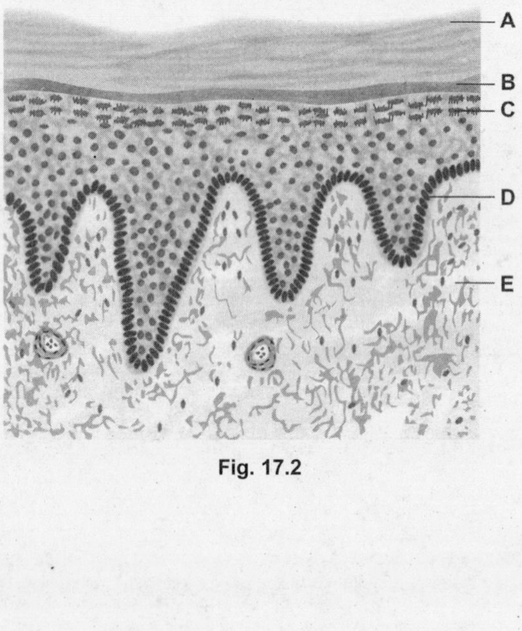

Fig. 17.2

Q3 **Figure 17.3 shows parts of hair follicle. Identify the parts.**

A. ____________________

B. ____________________

C. ____________________

D. ____________________

E. ____________________

F. ____________________

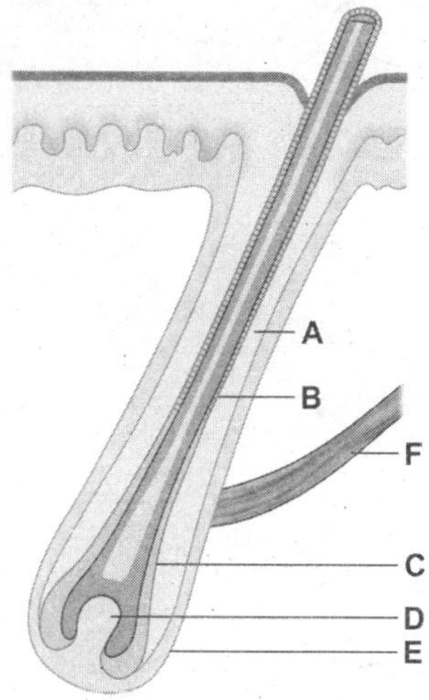

Fig. 17.3

Q4 **Draw a neat labelled diagram to show some important receptors present in relation to skin**

Q5 **Differentiate between thick and thin skin.**

Thick skin	Thin skin

Q6 **Differentiate between typical and atypical sweat glands**

Typical sweat glands	Atypical sweat glands

Q7 **Discuss briefly how body reacts and protects itself from cold.**

Q8 **Write short notes on:**

A. Functions of skin

B. Sebaceous glands

C. Tactile corpuscles of Meissner

D. Fever

Q9

Name the following:

A. Another name for stratum basale

____

B. The most superficial layer of epidermis

____

C. Cells producing melanin

____

D. Parts of body where glabarous/thick skin is present

____

E. Smooth muscle attached to hair follicle and dermis of skin

____

F. Secretion produced by sebaceous gland

____

G. Receptors for pain or discomfort

____

H. Part of brain playing important role in temperature regulation

____

I. Condition where body temperature falls below 35°C

____

Q10

Write True (T) or False (F):

A.	Thick skin has lot of hair	
B.	Skin is a highly vascular organ	
C.	Melanocytes are the predominant cell type in epidermis	
D.	Sebaceous and sweat glands are present in dermis of thin skin	
E.	Meibomian glands are modified sebaceous glands	

Q11

Match the following receptors with their respective sensation.

A.	Meissner corpuscle	1.	Pain
B.	Pacinian corpuscles	2.	Pressure
C.	Merkel cell endings	3.	Touch
D.	Nociceptors	4.	Vibration

CHAPTER

18

Introduction to Nutrition

Q1 **What are lifestyle disorders. Discuss briefly about obesity.**

Q2 **Define the following terms:**

A. Health

B. Macronutrients

C. Specific dynamic action

Q3 **Write short notes on:**

A. Malnutrition

B. Balanced diet

C. Basal metabolic rate

Q4 **Enlist:**

A. Micronutrients.

B. Diseases resulting due to vitamin deficiency.

C. Diseases resulting due to toxins in food.

D. Secondary causes of obesity.

E. Pathological conditions found more frequently in obese people.

F. Lifestyle disorders.

Q5 Write True (T) or False (F):

A.	Atherosclerosis is due to deposition of fat in arteries	
B.	An adult male requires 2000-2600 kcal of energy per day	
C.	Daily requirement of proteins is 1g/kg body weight	
D.	Android obesity is characterised by deposition of fat over waist area	
E.	Hypothyroidism and Cushing's disease are important endocrine causes of obesity	

Model Question Papers (Physiology)

MODEL QUESTION PAPER – I

Time : 2 Hours ***Maximum : 75 Marks***

SECTION A

I. Define erythropoiesis. Discuss the factors influencing it. Add a note on reticulocyte. Give a schematic representation of different stages of erythropoiesis. (2 + 5 + 3 + 3 = 13 marks)

II. Write short notes on:
a. Lung volumes and capacities
b. Second phase of deglutition
c. Arterial pulse
d. Juxtaglomerular apparatus (5 × 4 = 20 marks)

III. Write normal values of (including units)
a. Glomerular filtration rate
b. Duration of a cardiac cycle
c. RMP of a nerve
e. WBC count in an adult male (1 x 4 = 4 marks)

SECTION-B

IV. Name the hormones secreted from adrenal cortex. Describe the Physiological and Pharmacological actions of glucocorticoids. (3 + 7 = 10 marks)

V. Write short notes on:
a. Functions of thalamus
b. Organ of corti
c. Ovarian changes in menstrual cycle
d. Visual pathway and lesions
(5 × 4 = 20 marks)

VI. Name the following:
a. Lens used in the correction of astigmatism
b. Hormone responsible for milk ejection reflex
c. Vitamin playing significant role in blood coagulation
d. Abnormality due to increased growth hormone secretion after epiphyseal closure
e. Volume of air present in the lungs even after a forceful expiration
f. Macrophages present in liver
g. Hormone responsible for water reabsorption from the collecting ducts of kidney
h. A digestive enzyme present in saliva
(1 x 8 = 8 marks)

MODEL QUESTION PAPER-II

Time: 2 hours ***Maximum Marks: 75***

(Draw diagrams wherever necessary)

SECTION-A

I. Define blood pressure. Give its normal value. What is pulse pressure? Describe the mechanisms of regulation of blood pressure. (2 + 1 + 2 + 7 = 12 marks)

II. Write short notes on:
a. Factors affecting GFR
b. Digestion of carbohydrates
c. Immunity by T-lymphocytes
d. Active transport mechanisms (5 × 4 = 20 marks)

III. Write normal values of (including units)
   a. Platelet count
   b. Cardiac output in a young adult male
   c. Vital capacity in a young adult male
   d. PR interval (1 × 4 = 4 marks)

SECTION – B

IV. Name the sensations carried by posterior column fibers. With the help of a neat diagram, trace the pathway (4 + 7 = 11 marks)

V. Write short notes on:
   a. Indicators of ovulation
   b. Actions of insulin
   c. Functions of cerebellum
   d. Hypothyroidism (5 × 4 = 20 marks)

VI. Name the following:
   a. Neurotransmitter secreted by postganglionic sympathetic nerve fibers
   b. Hormone responsible for milk secretion
   c. Tract which transmits impulses for pain sensation
   d. Protein present in the thick filament of muscle fiber
   e. Ion responsible for pacemaker potential in cardiac muscle
   f. Lens used in the correction of hypermetropia
   g. Cells producing antibodies
   h. A hormone secreted from kidney
   (1 × 8 = 8 marks)

MODEL QUESTION PAPER – III

Total Marks : 50

1. Describe the mechanism of blood coagulation by extrinsic and intrinsic pathways. Add a note on hemophilia. (17 marks)
2. Explain the formation, circulation and functions of CSF. Add a note on blood-brain barrier. (15 marks)
3. Write short notes *on any three* of the following:
   a. Define
      1. Receptors
      2. Reflex
   b. Name four gastrointestinal hormones
   c. Functions of sertoli cells
   d. Functions of pancreatic juice (3 x 6 = 18)

MODEL QUESTION PAPER – IV

Total Marks : 50

1. Name the ascending tracts of spinal cord. Trace the pathway for pain, with the help of a neat, labelled diagram. (15 marks)
2. Define cardiac output. Give its normal value. What are the factors affecting it ? (17 marks)
3. Write short notes on :
   a. Functions of growth hormone
   b. Morphological classification of leukocytes and their functions
   c. Uterine changes during menstrual cycle.
   (3 × 6 = 18)

MODEL QUESTION PAPER – V

Total Marks : 50

1. Name the hormones secreted from anterior pituitary. Describe the functions of thyroid hormone. Add a note on its abnormalities. (17 marks)
2. What is the normal respiratory rate? Describe the chemical regulation of respiration. (13 marks)
3. Write short notes on :
   a. Spermatogenesis
   b. Tests for hearing
   c. Taste pathway
   d. Factors affecting glomerular filtration rate.
   (4 × 5 = 20)

MODEL QUESTION PAPER – VI

Total Marks : 50

1. Define blood pressure. Give its normal value. Describe the factors influencing it. Add a note on hypertension. (1 + 1 + 8 + 2 = 12)
2. Name the descending tracts of spinal cord. Describe the pyramidal pathway and its function. Differentiate lower motor neuron lesions from upper motor neuron lesions. (2 + 8 + 3 = 13)
3. Draw a labelled diagram of :
   a. Visual pathway
   b. Important cortical areas of brain (2 × 5 = 10)
4. Write the normal values of:
   a. Renal blood flow
   b. Vital capacity
   c. Sperm count
   d. Stroke volume
   e. Leukocyte count (5 × 1 = 5)
5. Write short notes on :
   a. Ovulation
   b. Rh incompatibility (2 × 5 = 10)

MODEL QUESTION PAPER – VII

Total Marks : 50

1. Describe the different phases of menstrual cycle and their hormonal background. (17 marks)
2. Draw a labelled diagram of the nephron. Give an outline of the process by which urine is formed. (15 marks)
3. Write short notes on :
   a. Normal spirogram
   b. Milk ejection reflex
   c. Functions of cerebellum
   d. Gastric juice
   e. Actions of testosterone
   f. Oral contraceptive pills (6 × 3 = 18 marks)

MODEL QUESTION PAPER – VIII

Total Marks : 25

1. Describe the process of erythropoiesis. Enumerate the factors affecting it. (7 marks)
2. Illustrate lung volumes and capacities. Discuss lung function tests. (3 + 4 = 7 marks)
3. Define blood pressure. Describe the factors affecting it. (5 marks)
4. Write short notes on any two. (3 × 2 = 6 marks)
   a. Placenta
   b. Ovarian cycle
   c. Intestinal motility
   d. Functions of liver
   e. Jaundice

MODEL QUESTION PAPER – IX

Total Marks : 25

1. Describe the intrinsic mechanism of blood coagulation. Mention the effect of heparin on it. (3 + 4 = 7 marks)
2. Discuss the physiological basis of artificial respiration. Add a note on acute oxygen toxicity. (3 + 4 = 7 marks)
3. Describe the movements of small intestine and discuss their neural control. (5 marks)
4. Write short notes on any two: (3 × 2 = 6 marks)
   a. Blood volume
   b. Micturition reflex
   c. Function of skin
   d. Milieu Interior
   e. Antidiuretic hormone

MODEL QUESTION PAPER – X

Total Marks : 25

1. Enumerate the chemicals regulating respiration. Describe the role of one of them. (3 + 4 = 7 marks)
2. Draw diagrams to illustrate
   a. Structure of eye
   b. Pathway for pain and touch (3 + 4 = 7 marks)
3. Discuss the factors affecting cardiac output (5 marks)
4. Write short notes on any two. (3 × 2 = 6 marks)
   a. Motor unit
   b. Function of hypothalamus
   c. Pain
   d. Middle ear
   e. Juxtaglomerular apparatus

Annexure

NORMAL VALUES (IN A HEALTHY YOUNG ADULT)

Blood, Formed Elements

Parameters	Normal values
pH of blood	7.4
Specific gravity	1.055–1.065
Osmotic pressure	290 milliosmoles/L
Viscosity	3.4–5.4
Plasma proteins	6.8 gm/100 ml
ESR	3-5 mm at the end of 1hour (in males) 5-12 mm at the end of 1 hour (in females)
PCV	45% (males) 42% (females)
Diameter of RBC	7.5 μm
RBC count	4.4–5.5 million/mm3 of blood (in males) 4-5 million/mm3 of blood (in females)
Hb	14–18 gm% (in males) 12–16 gm% (in females)
Total WBC count	4000–11,000 /mm^3 of blood
Differential count	Neutrophils: 50–70%, Basophils : 0–1%; Lymphocytes : 20-40% Monocytes : 2–8%
Platelet count	1.5–4 lakh/mm3 of blood

Respiratory System

Parameters	Normal values
Tidal volume	0.5 L (males), 0. 5 L (fmales)
Inspiratory reserve volume	3.3 L (males), 1.9 (females)
Expiratory reserve volume	1 L (males); 0.7 (females)
Reserve volume	1.2 L (males); 1.1 (females)
Total lung capacity	6 L (males), 4.2 L (females)
O_2 content in 100% saturated Hb	1.34 ml

Cardiovascular System

Parameters	Normal values
PR interval	0.12 to 0.2 sec
QRS duration	0.08 to 0.1 sec
QT interval	0.4 sec
ST segment	0.32 sec
Duration of cardiac cycle	0.8 sec
Cardiac output	5 L/min
Stroke volume	70 ml
End diastolic volume	130 ml
Blood pressure	120/80 mmHg
Heart rate	72/min

Urinary System

Parameters	Normal values
Renal blood flow	1.2 L/min
GFR	125 ml/min or 180 L/day
Renal threshold for glucose	180 mg/dL
Tubular maximum for glucose	375 mg/min
Urine output	1.5 L/day

Answer Key

Note: All the page numbers refer to the corresponding page of anatomy and physiology for nurses by Ashalatha fourth edition.

CHAPTER 1

1. **A.** Anatomical position; **B.** Supine position; **C.** Prone position; **D.** Lithotomy position
2. Refer page no. 4
3. **A.** Sagittal plane; **B.** Transverse plane; **C.** Coronal plane
4. **A.** Coronal suture; **B.** Sagittal suture; **C.** Lambdoid suture
5. **A.** Flexion; **B.** Extension; **C.** Abduction; **D.** Adduction; **E.** Medical rotation; **F.** Lateral rotation; **G.** Pronation; **H.** Supination; **I.** Inversion; **J.** Eversion; **K.** Opposition of thumb
6. **A.** Cranial cavity; **B.** Thoracic cavity; **C.** Abdominal cavity; **D.** Pelvic cavity
7. **A.** Right hypochondrium; **B.** Epigastrium; **C.** Left hypochondrium; **D.** Right lumbar; **E.** Umbilical; **F.** Left lumbar; **G.** Right iliac fossa; **H.** Hypogastrium; **I.** Left iliac fossa
8. Refer page no. 24
9. Refer page no. 10 and 11
10. Refer page no. 24
11. **A.** Refer page no. 5; **B.** Refer page no. 5; **C.** Refer page no. 7; **D.** Refer page no. 10
12. A–4; B–5; C–3; D–6; E–1; F–2
13. A–3; B–1; C–4; D–2
14. **A.** Superior (cranial); **B.** Inferior (caudal); **C.** Anterior (ventral); **D.** Posterior (dorsal); **E.** Superficial; **F.** Medial; **G.** Circumduction; **H.** Inversion; **I.** Ipsilateral; **J.** Reticuloendothelial system
15. A–4; B–1; C–5; D–2; E–3
16. **A.** False; **B.** True; **C.** True; **D.** False; **E.** True; **F.** True
17. **A.** Lateral; **B.** Inferior; **C.** Deep; **D.** Cranial cavity; **E.** Sign

CHAPTER 2

1. Refer page no. 28
2. Refer page no. 30
3. Refer page no. 31
4. Refer page no. 31 and Table 2.2
5. **A.** Refer page no. 28; **B.** Refer page no. 30; **C.** Refer page no. 33; **D.** Refer page no. 33; **E.** Refer page no. 32
6. **A.** True; **B.** True; **C.** False; **D.** False; **E.** True
7. **A.** Refer page no. 32; **B.** Refer page no. 32; **C.** Refer page no. 32
8. **A.** Dehydration; **B.** Polyunsaturated fatty acids; **C.** Scurvy; **D.** Isotopes; **E.** Calcium
9. A–2; B–4; C–1; D–5; E–3

CHAPTER 3A

1. Refer page no. 36
2. Refer page no. 40
3. **A.** Peripheral protein; **B.** Lipid bilayer; **C.** Transmembrane protein
4. Refer page no. 37, 38
5. **A.** Refer page no. 40; **B.** Refer page no. 41; **C.** Refer page no. 43; **D.** Refer page no. 41, 42; **E.** Refer page no. 40
6. Refer page no. 38
7. Refer page no. 39
8. **A.** Endoplasmic reticulum, Golgi complex, Mitochondria, membrane-bound vesicles; **B.** Microtubules, intermediate filaments, microfilaments; **C.** Simple diffusion, facilitated diffusion osmosis; **D.** Phospholipids and cholesterol. **E.** Nuclear membrane, nucleoplasm, nucleolus
9. **A.** Mitochondria; **B.** Nucleolus; **C.** Apoptosis; **D.** Centrosome; **E.** Brush border
10. **A.** Refer page no. 38; **B.** Refer page no. 45; **C.** Refer page no. 46; **D.** Refer page no. 46
11. A–4; B–1; C–2; D–5; E–3
12. **A.** True; **B.** False; **C.** True; **D.** True; **E.** False; **F.** False

CHAPTER 3B

1. Refer page no. 50
2. **A.** Refer page no. 52; **B.** Refer page no. 52; **C.** Refer page no. 52 and 53; **D.** Refer page no. 58 and 59; **E.** Refer page no. 58 and 59
3. **A.** Stratified squamous epithelium; **B.** Stratified cuboidal epithelium; **C.** Columnar epithelium showing cilia
4. **A.** Simple tubular; **B.** Simple coiled tubular; **C.** Unicellular; **D.** Simple branched tubular; **E.** Compound tubulo-alveolar
5. Refer page no. 61
6. Refer page no. 60, 61
7. **A.** Collagen fibers; **B.** Reticular fibers; **C.** Elastic fibers
8. Refer page no. 62
9. Refer page no. 68
10. **A.** Refer page no. 51; **B.** Refer page no. 62; **C.** Refer page no. 57
11. **A.** Tubular glands, acinar glands, alveolar glands; **B.** Trachea and large bronchi; **C.** Small intestine; **D.** Collagen fibers, reticular fibers, elastic fibers; **E.** Subcutaneous tissue, bone marrow, mammary gland, omenta and mesenteries, surrounding kidneys and behind the eyeballs
12. A–5; B–1; C–2; D–3; E–4
13. **A.** True; **B.** False; **C.** False; **D.** True; **E.** True

CHAPTER 4

1. **A.** Refer page no. 75; **B.** Refer page no. 80; **C.** Refer page no. 89; **D.** Refer page no. 93
2. Refer page no. 74, 75
3. Refer page no. 77, 78
4. Refer page no. 79 and 81
5. Refer page no. 75 and 76
6. Refer page no. 76
7. Refer page no. 80, 81
8. Refer page no. 82, 84
9. Refer page no. 86
10. Refer page no. 87
11. Refer page no. 94
12. Refer page no. 98
13. Refer page no. 98
14. Refer page no. 97

15. Refer page no. 84
16. **A.** Refer page no. 88; **B.** Refer page no. 94, 96; **C.** Refer page no. 90
17. **A.** Plasma; **B.** Buffy coat; **C.** RBC column
18. **A.** True; **B.** False; **C.** False; **D.** True; **E.** False; **F.** False; **G.** True; **H.** True; **I.** True; **J.** False; **K.** True
19. **A.** Pluripotent; **B.** Polycythemia; **C.** Anemia; **D.** Hemoglobin; **E.** Eosinophils; **F.** Fibrinogen; **G.** Prothrombin; **H.** Anticoagulants
20. **A.** 7.4; **B.** 1.7-2; **C.** Males – 4.5-5.5 million/mm^3, Females – 4-5 million/mm^3; **D.** Males – 14-18 g/100 mL, Females – 12-16 g/100 mL; Infants – 18-23 g/100 mL; **E.** Males – 40-45%, Females – 38-42%, **F.** 4000–11,000/mm^3; **G.** 1.5–4 lacs/mm^3

CHAPTER 5

1. Refer page no. 100
2. Refer page no. 101
3. Refer page no. 101
4. **A.** Area drained by right lymphatic duct; **B.** Area drained by thoracic duct
5. Refer page no. 103, Fig. 5.15
6. Refer page no. 108
7. Refer page no. 109
8. Refer page no. 110, 111
9. **A.** Pharyngobasilar fascia, palatoglossus muscle, superior constrictor muscle of pharynx; **B.** Jugulodiagastric mode, jugulo-omohyoid node, submental and submandibular nodes; **C.** Axillary lymph nodes; **D.** Inguinal lymph nodes; **E.** Splenic artery, splenic vein, efferent lymph vessels; **F.** Waldeyer's ring; **G.** Jugulodigastric lymph node; **H.** Splenomegaly; **I.** Spleen
10. Refer page no. 100
11. **A.** False; **B.** True; **C.** True; **D.** True; **E.** True; **F.** False; **G.** False; **H.** False

CHAPTER 6

1. Refer page no. 114, 115
2. Refer page no. 114, 115
3. **A.** Refer page no. 117; **B.** Refer page no. 118, 119; **C.** Refer page no. 119
4. Refer page no. 118
5. **A.** Refer page no. 118, 119; **B.** Refer page no. 116, 117
6. Refer page no. 118
7. **A.** True; **B.** True; **C.** False; **D.** True; **E.** False; **F.** True; **G.** True

CHAPTER 7

1. **A.** Cerebrum; **B.** Midbrain; **C.** Pons; **D.** Medulla oblongata; **E.** Cerebellum; **F.** Spinal cord
2. **A.** Dendrites; **B.** Nucleus; **C.** Axon hillock; **D.** Axon; **E.** Nissl bodies; **F.** Telodendria; **G.** Terminal boutons
3. **A.** Axon; **B.** Dendrite; **C.** Synaptic vesicles; **D.** Presynaptic membrane; **E.** Post synaptic membrane; **F.** Synaptic cleft; **G.** Mitochondrion
4. **A.** Latent period; **B.** Slow depolarization; **C.** Rapid depolarization; **D.** Rapid repolarization; **E.** After depolarization; **F.** After hyperpolarization
   A. –55 mV; **B.** +35 mV; **C.** To the opening sodium channels; **D.** To the closing of sodium channels and simultaneous opening of potassium channels
5. **A.** Anterior horn; **B.** Central part of lateral ventricle; **C.** Posterior horn; **D.** Inferior horn; **E.** Interventricular foramen; **F.** Third ventricle; **G.** Cerebral aqueduct; **H.** Fourth ventricle; **I.** Central canal
6. **A.** Frontal pole; **B.** Occipital pole; **C.** Median longitudinal cerebral fissure; **D.** Sulcus; **E.** Gyrus
7. **A.** Frontal pole; **B.** Temporal pole; **C.** Occipital pole; **1.** Central sulcus; **2.** Parieto-occipital sulcus; **3.** Posterior ramus of lateral sulcus
8. **A.** Anterior cerebral artery; **B.** Internal carotid artery; **C.** Middle cerebral artery; **D.** Posterior cerebral artery; **E.** Basilar artery; **F.** Posterior communicating artery; **G.** Anterior choroidal artery; **1.** Optic nerve; **2.** Optic tract; **3.** Optic chiasma
9. **A.** Claustrum; **B.** Putamen; **C.** Globus pallidus; **D.** Thalamus. **B and C** are collective called as lentiform nucleus
10. **A.** Substantia nigra; **B.** Crus cerebri; **C.** Middle cerebellar peduncle; **D.** Olive; **E.** Pyramid

11. **A.** Posterior median sulcus; **B.** Central canal; **C.** Substantia gelatinosa; **D.** Anterior median fissure; **E.** Anterior funiculus; **F.** Ventral gray column; **G.** Lateral gray column; **H.** Lateral funiculus; **I.** Dorsal gray column; **J.** Posterior funiculus; **K.** Posterior median septum. Refer page no. 165
12. **A.** Acetylcholine; **B.** Acetylcholine; **C.** Acetylcholine; **D.** Adrenaline or noradrenaline; **E.** Acetylcholine; **F.** Adrenaline or noradrenaline; **G.** Acetylcholine; **H.** Acetylcholine
13. Refer page no. 178. Fig. 7.67. The trochlear nerve is the only cranial nerve to emerge from dorsal surface of brain.
14. Refer page no. 133
15. Refer page no. 139. Fig. 7.21
16. Refer page no. 148. Fig. 7.34
17. Refer page no. 171. Fig. 7.63
18. Refer page no. 175. Fig. 7.66
19. Refer page no. 125. Fig. 7.3
20. Refer page no. 167. Fig. 7.56
21. Refer page no. 124. Flowchart 7.1
22. Refer page no. 126
23. Refer page no. 133, 134
24. **A.** Refer page no. 129; **B.** Refer page no. 133; **C.** Refer page no. 158; **D.** Refer page no. 166; **E.** Refer page no. 167; **F.** Refer page no. 176
25. **A.** Refer page no. 154, 155; **B.** Refer page no. 160; **C.** Refer page no. 175; **D.** Refer page no. 151; **E.** Refer page no. 153, 154
26. **A.** Refer page no. 131; **B.** Refer page no. 140; **C.** Refer page no. 140; **D.** Refer page no. 144, 145; **E.** Refer page no. 161; **F.** Refer page no. 168; **G.** Refer page no. 188; **H.** Refer page no. 195, 173
27. **A.** Refer page no. 177; **B.** Refer page no. 176
28. **A.** Astrocytes, microglia, oligodendrocytes, ependymal cells; **B.** Dura mater, arachnoid mater, pia mater; **C.** C-shaped choroidal fissures of lateral ventricles, roof of third ventricle, Roof of fourth ventricles; **D.** Pineal body, hypophysis cerebri, choroid plexus, median eminence; **E.** Midbrain, pons and medulla oblongata; **F.** Association fibers, projection fibers, commissural fibers; **G.** Caudate nucleus, lentiform nucleus, amygdaloid nucleus, claustrum; **H.** Feeding center and satiety center; **I.** Anterior cerebral artery and middle cerebral artery; **J.** Dorsal column tracts of Goli and Burdach or dorsal column fibers, anterior spinothalamic tract, lateral spinothalamic tract; **K.** Ventral rami of nerves C5-C8 and T1; **L.** Ventral rami of upper four lumbar nerves (L_1-L_4)
29. **A.** Oligodendrocyte; **B.** Schwann cell; **C.** Internode; **D.** Saltatory conduction; **E.** Third ventricle; **F.** Choroid plexus; **G.** Brainstem; **H.** Middle cerebellar peduncle; **I.** Clonus; **J.** Anesthesia
30. A–3; B–1; C–4; D–5; E–2
31. A–3; B–1; C–4; D–5; E–2

CHAPTER 8A

1. **A.** Perimysium; **B.** Epimysium; **C.** Endomysium
2. **A.** H-zone; **B.** Z-band; **C.** A-band; **D.** I-band; **E.** M-band in middle of H-zone
3. **A.** Axon terminal (motor end plate); **B.** Pre synaptic membrane; **C.** Post synaptic membrane; **D.** Synaptic cleft; **E.** Sarcoplasm
4. **A.** Cardiac muscle; **B.** Skeletal muscle fibers; **C.** Smooth muscle
5. **A.** Occipitofrontalis; **B.** Temporalis; **C.** Orbicularis oculi; **D.** Nasalis; **E.** Platysma; **F.** Orbicularis oris; **G.** Mentalis
6. **A.** Sterno cleido mastoid; **B.** Trapezius; **C.** Inferior belly of omohyoid; **D.** Posterior belly of digastric; **E.** Superior belly of omohyoid
7. **A.** Trapezius; **B.** Pectoralis major; **C.** Deltoid; **D.** Biceps; **E.** Brachialis; **F.** Brachioradialis; **G.** Flexor carpi radialis
8. **A.** Gluteus maximus; **B.** Biceps femoris; **C.** Semitendinosus; **D.** Gastrocnemius; **E.** Soleus; **F.** Calcaneal (achilles) tendon
9. Refer page no. 198-9
10. Refer page no. 202
11. **A.** Refer page no. 205; **B.** Refer page no. 201; **C.** Refer page no. 200; **D.** Refer page no. 205
12. Refer page no. 214
13. **A.** Refer page no. 207; **B.** Refer page no. 206
14. Occipitofrontalis – Refer page no. 209, Sternocleidomastoid – Refer page no. 211, Gastrocnemius – Refer page no. 232, Psoas major – Refer page no. 217, Deltoid – Refer page no. 221, Pectoralis major – Refer page no. 222, Latissimus dorsi – Refer page no. 223, Sartorius – Refer page no. 229

15. **A.** Psoas major, Psoas minor, Illiacus and Quadratus lumborum; **B.** Pectoralis major, pectoralis minor and lattissimus dorsi; **C.** Biceps brachii, brachialis and coracobrachialis; **D.** Gluteus maximus, medius and minimus; **E.** Adductor longus, adductor brevis, adductor magnus, pectineus, gracilis, and obturator externus; **F.** Masseter, temporalis, medial pterygoid and lateral pterygoid
16. **A.** Refer page no. 229; **B.** Refer page no. 203; **C.** Refer page no. 232; **D.** Refer page no. 217
17. Refer page no. 218
18. A–4; B–5; C–7; D–1; E–2; F–3; G–6
19. **A.** False; **B.** True; **C.** True; **D.** True; **E.** True; **F.** True; **G.** True; **H.** True

CHAPTER 8B

1. Refer page no. 237
2. **A.** Skull; **B.** Cervical vertebrae; **C.** Scapula; **D.** Sternum; **E.** Humerus; **F.** Radius; **G.** Ulma; **H.** Carpal bone; **I.** Metacarpals; **J.** Phalanges; **K.** Mandible; **L.** Clavicle; **M.** Ribs; **N.** Pelvis; **O.** Femur; **P.** Patella; **Q.** Tibia; **R.** Fibula; **S.** Tarsal bones; **T.** Metatarsals; **U.** Phalanges
3. **A.** Coronal suture; **B.** Sagittal suture; **C.** Lambdoid suture; **D.** Bregma; **E.** Lambda
4. **A.** Clavicle; **B.** Ribs; **C.** Scapula; **D.** Sternum
5. **A.** Body; **B.** Vertebral foramen; **C.** Pedicle; **D.** Transverse process; **E.** Spine; **F.** Superior articular facet; **G.** Superior costal facet
6. Refer page no. 239
7. Refer page no. 241
8. Refer page no. 243
9. Refer page no. 250
10. Refer page no. 260
11. **A.** Osteoblast, Osteoclast, Osteocytes and Osteoprogenitor cells; **B.** Ribs and sternum; **C.** Bones of skull, vertebral column, ribs and sternum. Hyoid bone is also the part of axial skeleton; **D.** Intramembranous or membranous ossification and endochondral or cartilaginous ossification; **E.** Clavicle, scapula, humerus, radius and ulna; **F.** Refer page no. 264; **G.** Sternocleidomastoid, Pectoralis major, Subclavius, deltoid and trapezius; **H.** Innominate/Hip bones (2 in number) and Sacrum and coccyx, **I.** Frontal, occipital, sphenoid, ethmoid, vomer and mandible, **J.** Refer page no. 254; **K.** First, second, tenth, eleventh and twelfth rib
12. **A.** Refer page no. 241; **B.** Refer page no. 238; **C.** Refer page no. 242; **D.** Refer page no. 260; **E.** Refer page no. 262-3; **F.** Refer page no. 280
13. **A.** False; **B.** True; **C.** True; **D.** True; **E.** False; **F.** True; **G.** False; **H.** True; **I.** True; **J.** False; **K.** True; **L.** False
14. A–3; B–5; C–1; D–2; E–4
15. **A.** Lambda; **B.** Mandible; **C.** Atlas; **D.** Foramen transversarium; **E.** Coccyx
16. A–3; B–4; C–5; D–1; E–2
17. **A.** Clavicle; **B.** Sternum; **C.** Humerus; **D.** Femur; **E.** Tibia and fibula

CHAPTER 8C

1. **A.** Articular cartilage; **B.** Fibrous capsule; **C.** Joint cavity; **D.** Periosteum; **E.** Synovial membrane; **F.** Synovial fluid
2. **A.** Ball and socket joint; **B.** Hinge joint; **C.** Pivot joint; **D.** Saddle joint
3. **A.** Dorsiflexion, 1. Refer page no. 300; **B.** Plantar flexion, Refer page no. 300
4. **A.** Flexion; **B.** Extension; **C.** Abduction; **D.** Adduction; **E.** Opposition
5. Refer page no. 284
6. Refer page no. 289-90
7. **A.** Refer page no. 285; **B.** Refer page no. 286; **C.** Refer page no. 286; **D.** Refer page no. 287; **E.** Refer page no. 291; **F.** Refer page no. 300–301; **G.** Refer page no. 286
8. A–3; B–1; C–4; D–5; E–2
9. **A.** Sternoclavicular joint and acromioclavicular joint; **B.** Subscapularis, supraspinatus, infraspinatus, teres major; **C.** Articular surface of the radius, articular disc of radio ulnar joint and scaphoid lunate and triquetral bone; **D.** Acetabulum of hip bone and head of the femur; **E.** Extension, flexion, medial rotation and lateral rotation; **F.** Refer page no. 302; **G.** Sutural joint, syndesmosis and gomphosis; **H.** Muscle producing inversion – Tibialis anterior and posterior, Muscle producing eversion – Peroneus longus and breuis
10. **A.** True; **B.** True; **C.** False; **D.** True; **E.** True

CHAPTER 9

1. **A.** Nasal cavity; **B.** Pharynx; **C.** Larynx; **D.** Trachea; **E.** Bronchi; **F.** Lung
2. **A.** Epiglottis; **B.** Hyoid bone; **C.** Thyroid cartilage; **D.** Cricoid cartilage; **E.** Trachea
3. **A.** Trachea; **B.** Primary bronchus; **C.** Secondary bronchus; **D.** Tertiary bronchus; **E.** Lobular bronchiole; **F.** Terminal bronchiole; **G.** Respiratory bronchiole; **H.** Alveolar duct; **I.** Alveolar sac
4. Refer page no. 317
5. Refer page no. 324
6. Refer page no. 308
7. Refer page no. 313
8. Refer page no. 320
9. Refer page no. 325
10. **A.** Refer page no. 307; **B.** Refer page no. 310; **C.** Refer page no. 320; **D.** Refer page no. 327; **E.** Refer page no. 329; **F.** Refer page no. 332
11. **A.** Refer page no. 324; **B.** Refer page no. 324; **C.** Refer page no. 324; **D.** Refer page no. 324; **E.** Refer page no. 325
12. **A.** Superior pulmonary vein, pulmonary artery bronchus with its vessels; **B.** Diaphragm and external intercostals; **C.** Scalene, sternodeidomastoids, neck and back muscles; **D.** Lateral cricoarytenoids, arytenoid; **E.** Recurrent laryngeal nerve, External laryngeal nerve; **F.** Upper lobe, middle lobe and lower lobe; **G.** Refer page no. 324; **H.** Refer page no. 307; **I.** Superior labial artery, anterior ethmoidal artery, posterior ethmoidal artery and branches of sphenopalatine artery; **J.** Carotid body and aortic body
13. **A.** False; **B.** True; **C.** True; **D.** True; **E.** False; **F.** True; **G.** False; **H.** True; **I.** False; **J.** True
14. A–2; B–3; C–1
15. A–2; B–4; C–1; D–3

CHAPTER 10A

1. **A.** Superior vena cava; **B.** Right pulmonary artery; **C.** Aorta; **D.** Left pulmonary artery; **E.** Right atrium; **F.** Inferior vena cava; **G.** Right ventricle; **H.** Left ventricle; **I.** Left atrium; **1.** Pulmonary valve; **2.** Tricuspid valve; **3.** Bicuspid valve; **4.** Aortic valve
2. **A.** Arch of aorta; **B.** Pulmonary trunk; **C.** Left auricle; **D.** Left ventricle; **E.** Left border; **F.** Apex; **G.** Right ventricle; **H.** Right atrium; **I.** Superior vana cava; **J.** Inferior vena cava
3. **A.** SA node; **B.** Internodal fiber; **C.** AV node; **D.** Bundle of His; **E.** Purkinje fibers
4. **A.** P wave; **B.** Q wave; **C.** R wave; **D.** S wave; **E.** T wave; **F.** PR interval; **G.** QRS complex; **H.** QT interval
5. Refer page no. 335-7
6. Refer page no. 334
7. Refer page no. 335
8. Refer page no. 336
9. Refer page no. 346
10. Refer page no. 344 and 353
11. Refer page no. 347
12. Refer page no. 356
13. **A.** Refer page no. 351; **B.** Refer page no. 354; **C.** Refer page no. 354; **D.** Refer page no. 350; **E.** Refer page no. 353; **F.** Refer page no. 348; **G.** Refer page no. 349
14. **A.** Refer page no. 352; **B.** Refer page no. 342; **C.** Refer page no. 357; **D.** Refer page no. 349; **E.** Refer page no. 349
15. **A.** Pericardium, myocardium and endocardium; **B.** Coronary sulcus; **C.** Apex beat; **D.** Sinoatrial node; **E.** Chordae tendinae; **F.** Refer page no. 342; **G.** Coronary sinus; **H.** a, c and v waves; **I.** Atrioventricular valves, semilunar valves
16. A–3; B–4; C–1; D–2
17. **A.** True; **B.** False; **C.** True; **D.** False; **E.** True

CHAPTER 10B

1. **1.** Arch of aorta; **2.** Ascending aorta; **3.** Thoracic aorta; **4.** Abdominal aorta; **A.** Right common carotid artery; **B.** Right subclavian artery; **C.** Right brachiocephalic artery; **D.** Right common iliac artery; **E.** Right internal iliac artery; **F.** Right external iliac artery

2. **1.** Falx cerebri; **2.** Out edge of tentorium cerebelli; **3.** Falx cerebelli; **A.** Superior sagittal sinus; **B.** Inferior sagittal sinus; **C.** Sphenoparietal sinus; **D.** Straight sinus; **E.** Transverse sinus; **F.** Occipital sinus; **G.** Sigmoid sinus; **H.** Great cerebral vein
3. **A.** Subclavian artery; **B.** Axillary artery; **C.** Brachial artery; **D.** Ulnar artery; **E.** Radial artery
4. **A.** Subclavian vein; **B.** Axillary vein; **C.** Brachial vein; **D.** Basilic vein; **E.** Cephalic vein; **F.** Median cubital vein; **G.** Median vein
5. **A.** Inferior mesentric vein; **B.** Superior mesentric vein; **C.** Splenic vein; **D.** Gastric vein; **E.** Portal vein; **F.** Cystic vein; **G.** Right and left branch of portal vein
6. **A.** Umbilical artery; **B.** Left umbilical vein; **C.** Portal vein; **D.** Ductus venosus; **E.** Inferior vena cava; **F.** Superior vena cava; **G.** Ductus arteriosus; **H.** Left pulmonary artery; **I.** Abdominal aorta; **J.** Inferior vena cava
7. Refer page no. 381
8. **A.** Refer page no. 360; **B.** Refer page no. 376; **C.** Refer page no. 367; **D.** Refer page no. 379-80
9. **A.** Tunica intima, Tunica media and Tunica adventitia; **B.** Brachiocephalic trunk, left common carotid artery and left subclavian artery; **C.** Refer page no. 365; **D.** Coeliac artery, superior mesentric artery and inferior mesentric artery; **E.** Retromandibular and posterior auricular vein; **F.** Radial artery and ulnar artery; **G.** Basilic vein, cephalic vein, median cubital vein and median vein
10. **A.** Brachiocephalic vein; **B.** Subclavian artery; **C.** Pectoralis minor; **D.** Brachial artery; **E.** Coeliac trunk; **F.** Inferior vena cava; **G.** Popliteal artery; **H.** Great saphenous vein
11. A–4; B–3; C–1; D–2
12. A–2; B–1; C–4; D–5; E–6; F–3
13. A–5; B–6; C–1; D–3; E–4; F–2
14. **A.** True; **B.** True; **C.** False; **D.** True; **E.** True; **F.** False; **G.** False; **H.** True; **I.** True; **J.** True

CHAPTER 11

1. **A.** Mouth; **B.** Pharynx; **C.** Esophagus; **D.** Liver; **E.** Pancreas; **F.** Stomach; **G.** Duodenum; **H.** Ascending colon; **I.** Transverse colon; **J.** Jejunum; **K.** Descending colon; **L.** Ileum; **M.** Sigmoid colon; **N.** Rectum; **O.** Anal canal; **P.** Caecum; **Q.** Appendix
2. **A.** Crown; **B.** Neck; **C.** Root; **D.** Enamel; **E.** Dentine
3. Refer page no. 390. Fig. 11.7
4. Refer page no. 403. Fig. 11.23
5. **Lobes: A.** Left lobe of liver; **B.** Quadrate lobe; **C.** Right lobe of liver; **D.** Cavdate lobe; **E.** Gall blader; **F.** Bare area;
   Ligaments: 1. Falciform ligament; **2.** Left triangular ligament; **3.** Right triangular ligament; **4.** Anterior coronary ligament;
6. Refer page no. 397
7. Refer page no. 405
8. Refer page no. 423
9. **A.** Refer page no. 389; **B.** Refer page no. 420; **C.** Refer page no. 402; **D.** Refer page no. 423; **E.** Refer page no. 398; **F.** Refer page no. 395
10. **A.** Refer page no. 389; **B.** Refer page no. 384; **C.** Refer page no. 395; **D.** Refer page no. 395; **E.** Refer page no. 409; **F.** Refer page no. 413; **G.** Refer page no. 419; **H.** Refer page no. 422; **I.** Refer Page no. 406
11. **A.** Refer page no. 395; **B.** Refer page no. 410
12. **A.** Mouth, oesophagus, stomach, small and large intestine, liver, gall bladder, rectum and anal canal; **B.** Duodenum, jejunum and ileum; **C.** Incisors, canines, premolars and molars; **D.** Fungiform, filiform pupillae, foliate and circumvallate; **E.** Nasopharynx, oropharynx and laryngopharynx; **F.** Parotid, submandibular and sublingual; **G.** Mucosa, submucosa, muscularis externa and serosa; **H.** Refer page no. 428-429; **I.** Refer page no. 426
13. Refer page no. 417-419
14. Refer page no. 405-407
15. **A.** Parietal cells of stomach; **B.** Common bite duct; **C.** Spiral valve of heister; **D.** Cholic acid and chenodeoxycholic acid; **E.** Hepato pancreatic ampula of Vater
16. **A.** Refer page no. 429; **B.** Refer page no. 429; **C.** Refer page no. 429; **D.** Refer page no. 430; **E.** Refer page no. 424
17. **A.** 4; **B.** 1; **C.** 2; **D.** 5; **E.** 6; **F.** 7; **G.** 3
18. **A.** 2; **B.** 4; **C.** 1; **D.** 5; **E.** 3
19. **A.** 3; **B.** 4; **C.** 1; **D.** 2
20. **A.** False; **B.** True; **C.** True; **D.** False; **E.** False; **F.** True; **G.** True; **H.** True; **I.** True; **J.** False

CHAPTER 12

1. **A.** Adernal gland; **B.** Kidney; **C.** Ureter; **D.** Urinary bladder; **E.** Renal artery
2. **A.** Renal cortex; **B.** Pyramid; **C.** Minor calyces; **D.** Major calyces; **E.** Pelvis
3. **(1) A.** Glomerulus; **B.** Proximal convoluted tubule; **C.** Decending limb; **D.** Loop of henle; **E.** Thin segment of ascending limb; **F.** Thick segment of ascending limb; **G.** Distal convoluted tubule; **H.** Collecting duct
   (2) Refer page no. 436
4. Refer page no. 441
5. Refer page no. 436
6. **A.** Refer page no 437; **B.** Refer page no. 439; **C.** Refer page no. 445
7. **A.** Refer page no. 437; **B.** Refer page no. 440; **C.** Refer page no. 443; **D.** Refer page no. 435
8. **A.** Glomerular filtration, tubular reabsorption, tubular secretion; **B.** Renal vein, renal artery, renal pelvis; **C.** Nephron is divided into renal corpuscle and tubular part. The renal corpuscle is divided into glomerulus and bowman's capsule and tubular part is subdivided into proximal convoluted tubule, distal convulated tubule and loop of henle; **D.** The capillary endothelium, Basement membrane, Foot process of podocytes; **E.** Juxtanglomerular cells, macula densa, Lacis cells
9. **A.** Refer page no. 441; **B.** Refer page no. 445; **C.** Refer page no. 443; **D.** Refer page no. 443; **E.** Refer page no. 446, 447
10. **A.** Refer page no. 442; **B.** Refer page no. 451; **C.** Refer page no. 444; **D.** Refer page no. 444
11. **A.** 3; **B.** 4; **C.** 1; **D.** 2
12. **A.** Proximal concentration tubule (PCT); **B.** Solutes with size more than 8 mm are not filtered, RBC, WBC and platelets; **C.** Atrial natriuretic peptide (ANP); **D.** Internal sphincter; **E.** Antidiuretic hormone (ADH)
13. **A.** True; **B.** True; **C.** False; **D.** False; **E.** True

CHAPTER 13

1. **A.** Short arm; **B.** Long arm; **C.** Secondary constriction; **D.** Centrosome; **E.** Primary constriction; **F.** Chromatid
2. **A.** Metacentric chromosome; **B.** Acrocentric chromosome; **C.** Submetacentric chromosome; **D.** Telocentric chromosome
3. Refer page no. 458
4. **A.** Refer page no. 456; **B.** Refer page no. 456, 460; **C.** Refer page no. 456; **D.** Refer page no. 459; **E.** Refer page no. 457; **F.** Refer page no. 458
5. **A.** Refer page no. 462; **B.** Refer page no. 464; **C.** Refer page no. 465
6. Refer page no. 465
7. **A.** 44 + XX; **B.** 44 + XY; **C.** 47 + XX; **D.** 45 + XO
8. Refer page no. 456
9. **1.** True; **2.** False; **3.** True; **4.** True; **5.** False; **6.** False; **7.** False; **8.** False; **9.** True; **10.** True

CHAPTER 14

FEMALE REPRODUCTIVE SYSTEM

1. **A.** Fallopian tube; **B.** Fundus of uterus; **C.** Uterine cavity; **D.** Body of uterus; **E.** Cervix; **F.** Vagina; **G.** Ovary; **X.** Broad ligament; **1.** Interstitial part; **2.** Isthmus; **3.** Amulla; **4.** Infundibulum with fimbriae
2. Refer page no. 473
3. Refer page no. 477. Fig. 14.11
4. Refer page no. 482
5. **A.** Refer page no. 478; **B.** Refer page no. 481
6. Refer page no. 484
7. Refer page no. 486
8. **A.** Outer serous coat or perimetrium, middle muscular coat or myometrium, inner mucus coat or endometrium; **B.** Isthmus; **C.** External os; **D.** Ovary; **E.** Stratified squamous epithelium; **F.** Anteverted and anteflexed; **G.** Stratum compactum, stratum spongiosum and stratum basale
9. **A.** Refer page no. 481; **B.** Refer page no. 486; **C.** Refer page no. 481; **D.** Refer page no. 479

10. **A.** Refer page no. 471; **B.** Refer page no. 475; **C.** Refer page no. 475; **D.** Refer page no. 476; **E.** 482
11. **A.** False; **B.** True; **C.** False; **D.** True; **E.** False; **F.** False
12. **A.** 3; **B.** 1; **C.** 4; **D.** 2
13. **A.** 2; **B.** 3; **C.** 1; **D.** 5; **E.** 4
14. **A.** 2; **B.** 1; **C.** 4; **D.** 3
15. **A.** 3; **B.** 4; **C.** 1; **D.** 2
16. **A.** 26 days; **B.** Progesterone; **C.** LH surge; **D.** Second polar body; **E.** 23X; **F.** Menarche; **G.** Round ligament; **H.** Progesterone

MALE REPRODUCTIVE SYSTEM

1. **A.** Seminal vesicle; **B.** Prostate gland; **C.** Urethra; **D.** Scrotum; **E.** Vas deferens; **F.** Epididymis; **G.** Testis
2. Refer page no. 496
3. **1.** Acrosomic cap; **2.** Proximal centriole; **3.** Basal body; **4.** Annulus; **5.** Axial filament; **A.** Head; **B.** Neck; **C.** Tail
4. **A.** Penis, scrotum, testis, epididymis and spermatic cord; **B.** Vas deferens or ductus deferens, seminal vesicle, ejaculatory duct, prostate, urethra; **C.** Spermatic cord; **D.** Tunica vaginalis, tunica albuginea and tunica vasculosa; **E.** Epididymis; **F.** Vas deferens
5. **A.** Refer page no. 494; **B.** Refer page no. 492; **C.** Refer page no. 497; **D.** Refer page no. 497
6. **A.** True; **B.** False; **C.** True; **D.** False; **E.** True; **F.** True; **G.** True; **H.** True

CHAPTER 15

1. **A.** Pituitary gland; **B.** Thyroid gland; **C.** Pineal gland; **D.** Parathyroid gland; **E.** Thymus; **F.** Adrenal gland; **G.** Pancreas
2. Refer page no. 501
3. **A.** Refer page no. 505; **B.** Refer page no. 506; **C.** Refer page no. 506; **D.** Refer page no. 511; **E.** Refer page no. 513; **F.** Refer page no. 519; **G.** Refer page no. 519; **H.** Refer page no. 523
4. Refer page no. 511
5. **A.** Refer page no. 501; **B.** Refer page no. 503; **C.** Refer page no. 515; **D.** Refer page no. 508–509
6. **A.** FSH, LH, TSH, ACTH, GH and prolactin; **B.** Vasopressin (ADH) and oxytocin; **C.** Thyroxine or tetraiodothyronine, tri-iodothyromine (T3) and calcitonin; **D.** Parathyroid hormone, calcitriol and calcitonin; **E.** Pars anterior, Pars intermedia, Pars posterior; **F.** Epiniphrine, Nor epinephrine and dopamine.
7. **A.** Hypophysis cerebri (pituitary gland); **B.** Hypothalamohypophyseal tract; **C.** Superior and inferior hypophyseal artery; **D.** Thyroid-stimulating hormone; **E.** Prolactin; **F.** Oxytocin; **G.** Antidiuretic hormone; **H.** Para follicular cells; **I.** Bones; **J.** Parathyroid hormone or parathormone; **K.** Zona glomerulosa of adernal cortex; **L.** Cushing's syndrome
8. **A.** 3; **B.** 5; **C.** 1; **D.** 2; **E.** 4; **F.** 6
9. **A.** True; **B.** True; **C.** True; **D.** False; **E.** True; **F.** False; **G.** True; **H.** False; **I.** True; **J.** True

CHAPTER 16

1. **A.** Auricle; **B.** External accoustic canal; **C.** Mastoid process; **D.** Styloid process; **E.** Tympanic membrane; **F.** Eustachian tube; **G.** Internal acoustic meatus
2. **A.** Tympanic membrane; **B.** Malleus; **C.** Incus; **D.** Stapes; **E.** Oval window; **X.** Tegmen tympani; **Y.** Tympanic cavity
3. **A.** Scala vestibuli; **B.** Scala media; **C.** Scala tympani; **D.** Spiral lamina; **E.** Membrana tectoria; **F.** Organ of corti; **G.** Basilar membrane
4. **A.** Scala vertibuli; **B.** Scala media; **C.** Scala tympani; **X.** Oval window; **Y.** Round window; **Z.** Aqueduct of cochlea.
   Fluid in **A.** Perilymph, **B.** Endolymph; **C.** Perilymph
5. **A.** Lacrimal duct; **B.** Conjuctival sac; **C.** Lacrimal gland; **D.** Lacrimal punctum; **E.** Lacrimal canalicus; **F.** Lacrimal sac; **G.** Nasolacrimal duct; **H.** Valve of Hasner
6. **A.** Cornea; **B.** Iris; **C.** Ciliary body; **D.** Sclera; **E.** Choroid; **F.** Retina; **G.** Fovea centralis; **H.** Optic nerve; **I.** Hyaloid canal; **J.** Lens
7. **A.** Refer page no. 531, Fig. 16.7; **B.** Refer page no. 539, Fig. 16.21; **C.** Refer page no. 530, Fig. 16.4; **D.** Refer page no. 551, Flowchart 16.3
8. **A.** Optic nerve; **B.** Optic chiasma; **C.** Optic tract; **D.** Lateral geniculate body; **E.** Optic radiation; **F.** Visual cortex
9. Refer page no. 550
10. **A.** Refer page no. 537; **B.** Refer page no. 537; **C.** Refer page no. 538; **D.** Refer page no. 548; **E.** Refer page no. 551

11. **A.** External ear, middle ear, internal ear; **B.** Malleus, incus, stapes; **C.** Superior rectus, inferior rectus, medial rectus, lateral rectus; **D.** Refer page no. 543; **E.** Refer page no. 545; **F.** Aqueous humor, vitreous humor; **G.** Rod and cones
12. **A.** 2; **B.** 3; **C.** 1
13. **A.** Taste buds; **B.** Elastic cartilage; **C.** Umbo; **D.** Internal jugular vein; **E.** Fovea centralis
14. **A.** True; **B.** False; **C.** False; **D.** True; **E.** True

CHAPTER 17

1. **A.** Epidermis; **B.** Dermis; **C.** Hair follicle; **D.** Sebaceous gland; **E.** Sweat glands
2. **A.** Stratum corneum; **B.** Stratum lucidum; **C.** Stratum granulosum; **D.** Stratum basale; **E.** Dermis
3. **A.** Outer root sheath; **B.** Hair root; **C.** Inner root sheath; **D.** Papilla; **E.** Bulb; **F.** Arrector pilli muscle
4. Refer page no. 562. Fig. 17.9
5. Refer page no. 557
6. Refer page no. 561
7. Refer page no. 564
8. **A.** Refer page no. 559; **B.** Refer page no. 560; **C.** Refer page no. 562; **D.** Refer page no. 564
9. **A.** Germinal layer or stratum germinativum; **B.** Stratum corneum; **C.** Melanocyte; **D.** Palm of hand and soles of feet; **E.** Arrector pili muscle; **F.** Sebum; **G.** Nociceptors; **H.** Hypothalamus; **I.** Hypothermia
10. **A.** False; **B.** True; **C.** False; **D.** True; **E.** True
11. **A.** 3; **B.** 4; **C.** 2; **D.** 1

CHAPTER 18

1. Refer page no. 574. For obesity refer page no. 571
2. **A.** Refer page no. 568; **B.** Refer page no. 569; **C.** Refer page no. 569
3. **A.** Refer page no. 571; **B.** Refer page no. 570; **C.** Refer page no. 569
4. **A.** Refer page no. 569; **B.** Refer page no. 570; **C.** Refer page no. 571; **D.** Refer page no. 573; **E.** Refer page no. 573; **F.** Refer page no. 574
5. **A.** True; **B.** True; **C.** True; **D.** True; **E.** True